"From an impoverished neighborhood of Boston to the surgical suites of one of the nation's most vaunted medical institutions, *Steep* recounts Craig Yorke's climb to become a respected neurosurgeon. A gifted violinist who might have filled a concert hall, he chose instead to exercise his virtuosity in caring for patients with neurosurgical disease. A complex story written with the same precision, clarity, and intensity that once guided his scalpel, *Steep* offers a rare window into the emotional and ethical terrain of a life spent on the front lines of life and death. It stands alongside the best medical memoirs—riveting, profound, and unforgettable."

—**Dr. Paul Camarata**
Chairman, Department of Neurosurgery and Chair, Neurosurgery, The University of Kansas Medical Center

"...a fascinating memoir by a distinguished Black neurosurgeon. But it is more than that; it's also evidence that professional achievement along with self-respect can bolster one's "armor" against racist condescension. A Boston Latin School and Harvard University graduate who received his surgical training in San Francisco, Dr. Yorke moved to Topeka, Kansas, to seize the opportunity to work with the renowned Menninger Foundation and to meet the community's need for a neurosurgeon. Dr. Yorke is a masterful storyteller."

—**Bill Tuttle**
Professor Emeritus of American Studies at the University of Kansas and the author of several books, notably including *"Daddy's Gone to War": The Second World War in the Lives of America's Children* and *Race Riot: Chicago in the Red Summer of 1919*

"Written with the deftness of a brain surgeon and the ear of a concert violinist, *Steep* is the unforgettably moving story of one man's life and times. But it is also a wise and courageous commentary on our time."

—**Cyrus Console-Soican, Ph.D.**
Professor of Liberal Arts, Kansas City Art Institute

"...skillfully woven into the times and places it describes, *Steep* takes the reader on a fascinating journey through diverse cultures and a transformative period in American history. His perspective is thoughtful and insightful. Ultimately, it's the compelling story of one person's life that illuminates a shared human experience of the times. Once I picked this book up, I didn't want to put it down."

—**Bryan Welch**
Author of *Beautiful and Abundant: Building the World We Want* & *The Gift of a Broken Heart: How Our Grief Can Connect Us*

"*Steep* is no less a profound meditation on the toll it takes to stand before the steep wall of lowering historical forces and the determination, discipline, and drive necessary in scaling it. What awaits at the summit, however, is unexpected; the ultimate reward of the author's journey upward is freedom—liberating self-knowledge and compassion for the struggles of others. *Steep* is about discovering what it is to become truly human. I can only hope that this, the author's first book, is not his last."

—**Tobias Schlingensiepen**
Member of the Kansas House of Representatives,
Senior Pastor First Congregational Church, Topeka, Kansas

"Using honest lessons gleaned at both the kitchen table and in the operating room, Dr. Yorke reflects on a life shaped by determination and choices made both for him and by him. In this compelling memoir, he shares powerful stories—offering a heartfelt look at the challenges and triumphs that define a life dedicated to healing."

−**Marsha Pope**
President Topeka Community Foundation

"...a compelling account of an unchartered climb from poverty to becoming a top neurosurgeon and the life lessons that have influenced and shaped the author. An inspiring must-read for anyone seeking encouragement and motivation on their life's journey, highlighting the transformative power of sharing our experiences."

−**Michael Kates**
History Teacher at Topeka Schools' Robinson Middle School, Kansas Teacher of the Year Nominee

---

"...a provocative book about Dr. Yorke's personal journey from childhood, adhering to his parents' dreams and plans for him, focusing on excellence in school, music, and athletic pursuits throughout childhood and his professional career. I found *Steep* a thoughtful reflection on life lessons and a compelling read."

−**Kathleen Sebelius**
44th Governor of Kansas, 21st U.S. Secretary of Health & Human Services

STEEP

A BLACK NEUROSURGEON'S JOURNEY

CRAIG YORKE

Flint Hills Publishing

Steep – A Black Neurosurgeon's Journey
© 2025 by Craig Yorke

All rights reserved. No part of this book may be reproduced, distributed, or transmitted in any form without written permission from the author, except in the case of brief quotations embodied in critical articles and reviews.

Cover Design by Amy Albright

Author Photograph by Ben Franklin, MD

Flint Hills Publishing
Topeka, Kansas
Tucson, Arizona
www.flinthillspublishing.com

Printed in the U.S.A.

Paperback Book: ISBN: 978-1-953583-98-7
Electronic Book ISBN: 978-1-966323-00-6
Hardcover Book ISBN: 978-1-966323-01-3

Library of Congress Control Number: 2024927490

On The Cover: Purkinje Cell, Human Cerebellum

These cells are among the most beautiful and easily recognized in the human brain, mimicking a minute oak tree. They were first revealed in the drawings of the Spanish artist and anatomist Ramon y Cajal in 1902, long before his microscopic images could be photographed. About 15 million of them live quietly, arrayed in tight formation at the bottom of our brains, and work to inhibit excessive muscle tone. They listen unceasingly to the world and our bodies through their thicket of millions of dendrites but speak only through a single transmitting axon. They keep our muscles balanced—neither too tight nor too loose, help us find our place in the world from one instant to the next. Right now, they are allowing the muscles of your arms and hands just enough contraction to hold this book still, and permitting your eyes to move accurately across these words. These are cautious inhibitory cells, conservative of energy. They favor stillness over action.

Conventional scientific wisdom in 1902 held that the human brain was a continuous network, but Cajal's drawings argued that it was composed instead of individual cells (about 100 billion). He suggested that those cells were separated by tiny spaces, decades before the electron microscope could see what we now call synapses. And, based purely on their architecture, he suggested that they communicated electrically, long before synaptic transmission could be detected. His work won a Nobel Prize in 1906 and the artistry of his pen and ink drawings launched the discipline we know today as neuroscience.

DEDICATION

To Zack and Chris

Ad astra per aspera

A Note to the Reader

I felt the impulse to write this book as I faced the Black Studies shelves of our local bookstore. It began as a letter to our sons. I marveled at the indisputable truth in those books, the scholastic rigor—pages brimming with courage, trauma, and righteous fury. Their diagnosis of America's racial illness was brilliant, the prognosis bleak. But I found little mention of treatment, and wondered where my story could find shelf space. I felt dwarfed by the forces they described, felt as powerless as any viewer of cable news. If these authors held the whole truth my life hadn't amounted to much. There was more to be said, value to be added.

Steep is my response to that bookstore moment. It isn't one more tale of winning against a stacked deck but a look at history's unspoken power through the lens of seven decades—at how the work of remembering can bring that power to light, can calm its voice.

The past shapes us all. Many flavors of tribal identity shrink our lives today, immunizing us against a sublime world brimming with surprise. *Steep* tells of waking up, of inching toward a more fluid self, toward some friendship with that past—and so toward some space for the future.

Craig Yorke
April 2025

The great force of history comes from the fact that we carry it within us, are unconsciously controlled by it.

—James Baldwin

CONTENTS

Stealth
-1-

Crucible
-15-

Educated
-39-

The Better Angel
-63-

Fledgling Pillars
-83-

Peaks and Valleys
-101-

Twilight of Expertise
-127-

New Eyes
-149-

-1-
STEALTH

I lifted the phone on its first ring and ordered the usual studies. It perched about 18 inches from my left ear and seldom brought good news after midnight. My new patient had run his motorcycle into a tree. He'd been unhelmeted and was now deeply unconscious. The ER told me the ambulance would reach them in about 15 minutes.

I swung my legs left and stood. Neurosurgery was my day job, a practice humming with variety. I also covered Topeka's hospitals and the surrounding region every other night and every other weekend. These calls weren't infrequent. My beeper, wallet, and keys were in their usual places by the bathroom sink, my clothes draped on the door's hook. The drive to the ER took five minutes. No need to speed—the roads were empty.

He and I arrived together. Unnumbered fragments of gravel, glass, and dirt were embedded in his face and arms. A cervical collar placed in the field protected his spinal cord. Bleeding from the scalp had slowed but his blond mane was matted with clot. He didn't move or resist the presence of the plastic tube in his windpipe. The smells were routine for that hour in that little, brilliantly lit cubicle—alcohol seasoned liberally with blood and vomit. A urine drug screen would reveal he'd made serious efforts to alter his mind.

I moved toward the gurney as the nurse began shearing off his T-shirt. She stopped just short of his collar, recoiled, hissed. I glanced up to see the tattoo covering his chest. The block letters proclaimed: "WHITE POWER."

Our family lacked power in 1950. Our tribe did not hold the high ground. Mom and Dad's struggle was hardly unique, and combat had begun long before I could name the enemy. Could it have been the smiling baker next door, who had chosen that afternoon to repaint his shop? Probably not. Or the battalion of roaches who migrated from his bakery later that night in search of better air, migrated through my nursery and into my crib, only to be driven back into the dark by my parents' frenzy? And what devil had tempted me a few days later to crawl behind our refrigerator to enjoy bread intended for rats? I recall the desperate sprint to Boston City Hospital only as family lore but recoil at the smell of Ipecac to this day.

These memories live. And they do not age. Baldwin's words greet every visitor at the entrance to the National Museum of African American History and Culture. As I sit with my own past, I confront the control he describes and am reminded that my imperfect memory mixes literal with psychological truth, curating the experience and bending the chronology. Blame fades and time runs. I'll say here what cannot be fully conveyed at Thanksgiving dinners. What somehow doesn't come up on family vacations. Will chronicle the price and the value of success. Will get close to what hurts.

Begin with my folks, Dorothy and Craig, Sr. Mom and Dad loom large in this telling because I arrived as they prepared to adopt after seven years of childless marriage, also because I was sickly, struggling with asthma and a clubbed right foot. And crucially, because they had neither money nor fertile time for a second child, making of me one miraculous, fragile, solitary, and heavily-scrutinized kid.

Dad was born in 1912 in New Bedford, Massachusetts, the oldest of three boys. His family had lived in that old whaling town for three generations and enjoyed some local prominence. His grandfather's family had more than once welcomed Frederick Douglass as a house guest. His parents, Everett and Carrie, defied middle class mores by divorcing in 1917 and rejected adulthood by insisting that neither would accept custody of their boys. They were placed at St. Mary's Home, a local Catholic orphanage when my dad was five, his brothers three and two. Everett and Carrie would visit from shouting distance on the occasional Sunday, waving to their

STEEP

sons through the Home's wrought iron fence.

Dad was soon diagnosed with tuberculosis and transferred to Sasquatcham Sanitarium, joining other TB patients and soldiers recovering from chlorine gas exposure in the trenches of France. He found himself alone and suddenly an adult in Boston at age 12, taking on more than his share of rough edges. He first learned at 14 that he had two brothers, and legally changed his last name at about age 20 to voice his opinion of his parents, declaring himself without family, no longer York but Yorke. Their desertion shaped him. He looked for explanations, but the answers shifted over time and failed to satisfy. His own dad's boundless self-regard had birthed a combative and suspicious kid. He embodied every reflex of the streets but was fanatically determined to chase legitimate success.

Mom was born in Newport News, Virginia in 1918 and came to Boston the next year when her family joined the Great Black Migration north for work and respect. Her dad, John, was a genial man who found occasional work as a barber but more reliable solace in his bourbon. Her mom, Lavinnia, grimly anchored the family by default, working in joyless domestic service for a parade of imperious women.

As Mom grew up, she found her suitors to be noisy, quick to posture but slow to act, comfortable with their assigned places in the social order. Neighborhood parlance named them Four Flushers. That they were janitors or laborers had been decreed by their color, but their comfort with the edict rankled. She often recalled one as beautiful to look at, a man made entirely of fabric—an empty suit. She saw the fires that fueled my dad. He saw a chance to win a beautiful woman and join a less fractured family. They first took serious note of each other in 1940 on a frozen Charles River where he taught her to skate. She later taught him to swim, a far more challenging task. He proposed marriage on their first date.

They were eager to overturn the verdict of their own history. They courted in Boston's ghetto, where their outsized ambitions regularly collided with reality. This was a grim place; the Harlem renaissance didn't reach so far north. The city had long had its no-go neighborhoods. And the racial climate was severe long before mandated school busing dragged the city into national news in the 1970s. Boston's supporters linked its downtown landmarks in 1951 to create the Freedom Trail. It has inspired generations of tourists but was a bitter oxymoron for the young lovers. They tallied every slight without public retort and lived as secret agents, invisible long before Ralph Ellison picked up his pen.

But America's lid was being pried off as I arrived in 1948. Harry Truman had integrated the armed forces. Joe Louis and Jackie Robinson were points of pride. Almost 60 years earlier in Atlanta, the public intellectuals W.E.B. DuBois and Booker T. Washington had debated the best way forward for Black folks. Washington had argued for nurturing a generation of yeoman farmers and small businessmen, a parallel society patient in its ambitions and barricaded against the worst of America. DuBois found that idea craven, its advocates too ready to accept Jim Crow as permanent. He imagined that a few intellectuals, a "talented tenth," could better lead the race and secure its rightful place in a diverse modernizing nation. He discarded that idea the year I was born.

But Mom and Dad were passionate DuBois fans and had no doubt that their son would be among that elect. I would be their stealth weapon, their guided missile to atomize the world's contempt, would lead the life they had been denied. Or, if not a missile, an adamantine shield forged to deflect every insult. Parents routinely assure their kids that they can achieve anything, words of hilarious gibberish for my ancestors. But now history was pivoting and our household's hunger for recognition would be difficult to overstate. I'd been born at the right time, the perfect time, and surely must outperform. I must become what they and their peers named a credit to the race, must live in service to the cause. So—they held me close and guarded me well.

I was conceived in December 1947 on the third floor of 218 West Canton Street, a brownstone in Roxbury, Boston's Black ghetto. Mom and Dad had sublet space from her parents, but money was tight. Their friends would sometimes chip in to gather in that space, affairs known since the 1920s as rent parties. After his TB test kept him from active duty, Dad worked as a laborer at the Hingham shipyard south of Boston. A string of night school courses and a wartime shortage of white men allowed him to break in as a draftsman in 1945. The process was contentious, the words "break in" intended. His college career at Lincoln University, a Black school in Pennsylvania, had been foreclosed in 1931 after a single semester for lack of tuition money. Mom was proud of her own degree from Boston Clerical School and of her work as a private secretary. She had intimate knowledge of her Smith Corona and its temperamental ribbons.

West Canton Street had gentrified dramatically by 2003 when I took Dad back for an East Coast roots trip. He unfolded himself from our compact rental car, waved his black walnut cane at the block of now elegantly restored brownstones and regaled me with tall tales of the neighborhood. He agreed that the old place had been beautifully maintained but when I told him that its value had grown more than 40-fold, he responded with stunned silence followed closely by colorful expressions of disbelief.

The neighborhood was gritty, of course, but very much alive, birthing more than its share of admirable Americans. One of them came to the aid of my Aunt Mabel, dad's brother's wife, in May 1945. Her labor had begun unexpectedly, giving her an urgent need for a ride to Boston Lying-In Hospital. Wartime gasoline rationing and racial economics had thinned the traffic. And ambulances were slow to reach Roxbury. But she had heard of a young man with a car, only a few houses away. Malcolm Little was ready to help. He and his car saved the day. He needed that car for business, the business of burgling suburban houses on weekend nights. He enjoyed a high profile in Roxbury and drew police attention barely a month later. While in the Charles Street Jail for armed robbery, Mr. Little educated himself by transcribing Webster's entire dictionary—from aardvark to zyzzya—and later changed his last name to X. Meanwhile, Mabel's son Bryant, my cousin, was safely delivered and became a professor of computer science and my good friend. Malcolm was a complex figure, but part of him for me lives in memory as a compassionate red-haired youngster.

Mom's labor began as she and Dad roasted in the Fenway Park bleachers late in the afternoon of August 19, 1948. He suppressed his panic and got moving. Traffic was heavy and stress was high. I was born long haired and loud, privileged to be delivered not in Roxbury but in nearby Jamaica Plain, and by a white obstetrician. My club foot was a nasty surprise, its bottom turned fully in rather than down.

Our family soon moved to an apartment on 99 Waumbeck Street. Our new neighbors were less desperate and included a smattering of Jews. But the bankers' red lines still corralled us all. The family lore of roaches and rat poison flows from that address, its hard realities pushing us to move on.

In 1953 we migrated to Dorchester, another of Boston's neighborhoods, reaching for a slice of the American dream to buy an aging Victorian house on Brunswick Street. I bounced my tricycle over the oak tree roots in the front yard and would walk only a few minutes through a field of lilacs and ragweed to reach Grandma Lavinnia's house on Intervale Street. That field, a vacant lot in the eyes of any adult, was a vast and mysterious savannah for this five-year-old. We three would make our way across that field for elaborate holiday dinners and encounter an array of maternal aunts, uncles, and cousins.

I was once enlisted to carry a covered dish of creamed green beans across that field, to keep it level at all costs. I was relieved to succeed, and squeezed our contribution onto a dining table already sagging under the weight of spectacular soulful food. I heard raucous debates among the menfolk about who was the better athlete—Joe Louis or Jackie Robinson. Or which car, Lincoln or Cadillac, carried greater prestige. I'd already been well enough closeted that I couldn't quite penetrate my cousins' jokes and secrets. And Grandma threatened to "beat the black" off us if we misbehaved.

Lavinnia was a short, thick woman, fashioned from some indestructible material, a taciturn, reluctant anchor for us all. She was forever host, never guest. During those many celebrations I recall her smiling only once—at some mysterious adult yarn. There were endless debates about skin and hair, an intricate and subtle reckoning of caste. Her house was filled with boisterous laughter. But amid all the debating and feasting the adults did agree on one point—that we were all perpetually despised, untouchable. What else to conclude from movies, newspapers, from the Church and the State? We faced a full court cultural press, were suffocated by a totalitarian condemnation.

Yet within our tribe there were infinite distinctions. My hair could be improved by liberal application of grease and a too tight nylon stocking cap, but my skin was problematic. In winter it was barely darker than a paper bag, offering conditional entry into more elite circles. But summer reliably tanned me an unacceptable chocolate. Mom made a desultory effort to keep me indoors and retard the sun's effect. That impulse was futile, but she did forbid me from reminding the world of my color by wearing anything brown. Red was beyond the pale.

Many years later I was in Boston for a meeting and had an impulse to revisit Intervale Street. I hailed a taxi and asked to go to Grandma's old address. The driver, jet-black Sudanese, bluntly refused and ordered me out of his cab. I told him a bit about my family history and negotiated an agreement. That we were speaking at the entrance to an overpriced downtown hotel in broad daylight was in my favor. He agreed to drive to the address and wait two minutes with his motor running if I promised not to exit the cab.

The street and its history were alive and well in my memory, but when we arrived, I recognized nothing of the blasted landscape. Black iron bars defended the few unbroken windows, and exuberant weeds were gradually uprooting the sidewalks. Mounds of garbage testified to habitation, but no one was to be seen. He said something about a crack war, and I didn't need my full two minutes. On our return ride he preached that the lazy people of Intervale Street had much to learn from industrious African immigrants like himself. The torrent of his words flooded the cab's cabin, and I had no appetite for debate with this strident zealot. Part of me had been stolen, recovered in a disfigured state.

That first home on Brunswick Street was a major point of pride, its mortgage an emblem of American inclusion. I ventured into the first grade just around the corner at the Atherton School on Columbia Road. But I wasn't faring well in playground combat. And a brothel had moved in across the street from our new home. One October afternoon I came home trickling blood from a puncture wound in my right calf. Under interrogation I told Mom a girl had stabbed me with her pencil during recess. We both could see the fragment of lead under my skin. Mom pulled out her tweezers and sewing needles, struck a match to sterilize her instruments, and wiped my skin with mercurochrome. She silently levered the needle under her target as I wailed. It wriggled away from her tweezers again—and again. Now we were both in real pain. She finally gave up and I breathed. She ruminated for weeks about lead poisoning.

I was struggling to read too, just as a few suburban schools were introducing a new teaching tool called phonics. So—we moved again, this time to Stoughton, a white working-class town 20 miles southwest of the city. A radical and consequential decision in 1954. Mom's family worried enough about the mortal danger posed by this alien enclave that her older brother quietly offered my dad a revolver. Dad knew violence well. He and Mom knew their risk, but the offer brought it home, focused their attention. Mom often said they'd talked through the dangers, but I never learned whether they'd accepted the weapon. My best guess today is that Dad knew his temper well enough to turn it down.

We were emigrating from their community and their secure place within it. Old photos show them with attractive, stylish peers. Dad was a Mason and belonged to the Omega Psi Phi fraternity. Mom modeled for NAACP fashion shows. But they lived at the margins of this Black Bourgeois. Dad lacked family, felt he had no "people"—his lack of a college credential gnawed at his self. They aimed less to socialize than to rise. And now they were displacing themselves, maybe into harm's way, in exchange for a hope in the unseen and for their son's shot at literacy.

The GI Bill had filled Stoughton with ethnicities from all over Europe. Mom, who looked white, handled all our home buying and selling. Dad's color would have aborted any transaction. He accepted this fact without comment, at least to me. Family from both sides visited our little ranch house outpost at first, less often as time passed. Dad was exquisitely attentive to who ate too much or failed to reciprocate our hospitality. The nuclear family tightened—and my future narrowed. Our emigration and the upward mobility they craved would carry a cost for them, a higher price for me. I wonder how carefully they had weighed their move.

I did learn to read. I read *Think and Do*, a second-grade workbook, and remember my teacher wearily telling my parents that I much preferred doing to thinking. I tasted childhood, playing long afternoons in a nearby forest and in a contractor's giant sandlot across from our house. Dad taught me how to shovel heavy wet snow that first winter—bent knees, straight back, gentle twist, no hurry. He took pains with his technique and his rhythm. Men died each winter doing this task—one just down the street had been 52 years old.

We fished once, sat at the shore of a tiny pond on a still Saturday morning. My relentlessly kinetic Dad did not speak or move. I mirrored him. A fish found my hook. I had succeeded without effort! But this tiny perch insisted on life. It jumped out of my bucket, kept jumping along the shore. Its scales cut my hands as I tried to recapture it. Its taste did not satisfy. All this fishing and shoveling aimed for a normal boyhood in an alien town.

My stiff royal blue shirt proclaimed me a real Cub Scout as I wolfed down Pecan Sandies after our first meeting. We gathered in a church basement fellowship hall. Behind the scoutmaster an American flag (with 48 stars) nearly covered the wall. Our young voices rendered the national anthem with more spirit than skill, but my career ended soon after Mom likened our troop to a Hitler Youth squadron. I enrolled in Little League Baseball.

Dad had played for the Philadelphia Colored Giants and was

quick to mention that he had managed a hit off Satchel Paige (years later he confided that it had been a successful bunt). He was now my fanatical instructor. He'd kept his glove from those years, a single thickness of mahogany brown cowhide with five bulbous peninsulas for thumb and fingers. For me it was a small animal, a kind of leathery crab, smelling of the saddle soap he used each spring to keep it supple. For him it was more old friend than tool, an unpadded mitt barely larger than his calloused, practiced right hand. He parted with it reluctantly late in life, a casualty of one of his many changes of address—I'm poorer for his choice. He struggled to be patient with his eight-year-old student, and I found endless ways to disappoint.

My clubbed right foot was certainly an obstacle to athletic success, turned inward enough to make me more tortoise than hare. They'd been well advised against surgery and had instead chosen a treatment featuring daily exercises and clunky corrective shoes I wore till I was 12. My physical therapist was persistent, as gentle as she was skillful. Dad designed a therapeutic device, a heavy elastic band linking a stout leather loop sewn onto the outer side of my right shoe to a heavy bandage on my outer thigh, persistently tugging my foot toward normalcy. The elastic was as thick as my thumb and the thigh bandage was held in place with three layers of thick adhesive tape—a creative and loving splint.

Pulling that tape off every few days provoked a reliable flow of tears. I was certain that this ordeal would be permanent, whatever Dad's reassurances. I so wanted to run with the other kids, to wear normal shoes, wanted to belong. I don't remember what else I felt about my condition or its treatment but know that whatever feelings I expressed would have been irrelevant, actually unheard. Dad took charge of the dressing changes, reminding me at each encounter to be a big boy and quit crying, calling for my Y chromosome to assert itself.

Reading and writing were fundamental to the bulletproof kid my folks were raising, but cultural literacy was indispensable too. They aimed for discipline, restraint, persistence. I was to learn something hard, something that most kids didn't. So, violin lessons began at age seven. I was a reluctant student, once broke my undersized bow in anger and paid for it with many weeks of allowance. One nickel per week.

Their scrutiny was undivided, their knowledge of a hostile world was beyond my childish imagination. Their loving severity would prepare me for what they knew that world had in store. I was to do as I was told, to "get ready." No surprise that my memories of talking back are few. I was a busy kid, but endured many anxious afternoons in my tiny bedroom after hearing "wait till your father comes home" echo in my ears. And I do remember being spanked. Often.

Mom would insist that I had been a willful child. I sensed that we were in hostile territory but couldn't fathom the grownups' rules of engagement. I did fight a lot with other boys over boyish things, fought in the schoolyard and in the neighborhood, fought to be part of a family at war with the world, leaving my folks furious if I lost and terrified if I won. Dad shared a few street fighting moves with me but the lessons were hard to recall when they mattered most. We had publicly joined the town. Mom worked in the PTA and Dad even won a local election and became a selectman. But countless kitchen table homilies conveyed a darker reality. Our new home was free of rats and roaches, but this America I would confront was relentlessly hostile and to be navigated entirely alone. I must be competent beyond all criticism, despised but unrejectable, must weather its contempt, whether rabid or serene. The Irish were our particular villains. The survivors of the potato famine now held power in local business and politics, were the police who reminded us of our place. They of course had suffered decades of British bigotry and now we were the victim's victim.

My parents had attended countless community meetings, signed petitions, canvassed for many politicians back in the city, but were now impatient with the pace and intrigues of the local Civil Rights Movement, despairing that "our people will never get it together." So, they began to carve a solitary path for themselves and for me.

By 1959, Dad had taught himself to be an electrical engineer and was commuting to a job in Boston. Years later his hard-won professional certificate would hold its place of honor on our living room wall. So now we moved yet again, to a tiny apartment at 80 Corey Road in Brighton, a more mixed Boston neighborhood. The move meant a shorter commute for him and a local address that would let me apply to a special public school for the 7th grade. They were deferring gratification across decades now, expressing their tenacious brand of love. I was to live the life they'd been denied. My role as surrogate would soon intensify.

First, though, came sixth grade, one block north of our apartment, at the Harriet A. Baldwin School. Kevin Sullivan became my friend there. He was a sportsman, converting our living room sometimes into a baseball diamond, sometimes a boxing ring. His elvish energy was a delight, and he was welcome in our home despite his ethnicity. But the walls of our bunker slowly separated me from likely friends. The distance grew with time. There were days I felt I was in school by myself. Kevin was one of so many I've lost touch with. Ironically, he found our apartment palatial since he lived in a brutal public housing project four blocks away.

Saturday mornings featured Dad's pancakes drenched in maple syrup, a craving that follows me to this day. The refined sugar was a reliable refuge from the world's expectations. The well-used gray Formica kitchen table harbored pancake fragments and bits of sticky syrup deep in its cracks and divots long after breakfast was over. We cleaned that table and much else with generous doses of Comet. Fumes from the oil furnace in the basement seasoned our winter meals. The black and white linoleum covering the kitchen floor had been sized in haste by an indifferent landlord. It wriggled under our feet as we walked, its edges rolling an inch or two up the walls.

Dad struggled to readapt to city life, defending his street parking space with hard words and credible threats, especially after we'd shoveled it in winter. My new bedroom was smaller, the neighbors closer, the sun more distant. Sunday afternoons were for music—Ella Fitzgerald to Jascha Heifetz, Errol Garner to Mahalia Jackson. The Sunday *New York Times* shaped our politics and the *New Yorker* our aspirations. Their cartoons offered a welcome respite in a household short on humor.

Our quarters were tight, but I remember little intimacy between my parents, only seamless teamwork. Public displays of affection did not happen. Dad was often volcanic but could reliably bring himself to attend to Mom's voice when it mattered most. They faced the same humiliations as every other Black American, but they didn't despair or self-immolate. They met insult not with angry rhetoric, but with mundane action, day after day. They trusted that their climb would bring relief, made themselves outliers and me with them. They loved each other as they loved their 11-year-old, loved as they could, their affection yoked to a bottomless craving for the world's respect.

I played close by at Dean Park or at the Baldwin schoolyard but was the only kid out there with a wristwatch. I'd lose an afternoon outside for every five minutes I was late getting home. My boyish playground adventures and fantastic explorations were all very well but also well beside the point. Being late—indulging in "colored people's time"—simply could not happen.

Michel Sasson became my new violin teacher. He played in the Boston Symphony, had been born in Egypt, and educated in Paris. His own training at the conservatory there had been merciless, and his severity was a shock to me, but Mom (who took notes at every lesson for the next six years) fully approved. I certainly didn't play well in those early years. The noise I made was hard even for me to endure. But there was no alternative to practicing at least two hours each afternoon. Improvement did come but was too slow for me to perceive. Tenacity underpinned this campaign for upward mobility and the violin was a core tool. I did play well at one lesson in about 1964, a hint of things to come. Sasson closed my book and assigned the next week's work, muttering, "I have nothing to say." Mom nodded with delight.

I was a sixth grade athlete. Our Baldwin basketball team scored an improbable win one December night against a much better squad from a nearby school. I was far more skillful at fouling than rebounding or shooting, but I remember the intoxicating team spirit and the bitter cold as we left that gym, pushing clouds of gray vapor into the still night air. I also said goodbye to my corrective shoes the next July. The exercises and taping had done their work over what felt like geologic time. I should remember some sort of celebration but don't. I was running from the past, thirsting for the future—and missing a peak moment of my boyhood. The present was not a place for us to linger. My new pair was no less sensible, and cheaper.

I played my last Little League Baseball game that summer at Cleveland Circle Park, close to home. Dad helped coach the team. He knew far more about the game than any of the other dads and was quick to say so. He won no popularity contests. I was tall for my age and opposing coaches often questioned my eligibility. I remember my birth certificate being trotted out more than once. He was desperate for me to succeed and loudly annoyed with his 11-year-old's attention span, but taught me well. I ultimately became a star player, making good use of my new right foot. I remember once hitting a home run, far over the center fielder's head, and was amazed at the flight of the ball. All his advice had been sound—weight transfer, hip rotation, level swing, still head. No sting in my hands, just as he had predicted. He was triumphant that afternoon and for years would recount every detail of the event to anyone who would stay still. I was at first embarrassed, later at peace with his limitless pride. He felt I had talent, but Mom insisted it was time to put away childish things. No call for more Black runners and jumpers. No more baseball.

-2-
CRUCIBLE

"The past is never dead. It's not even past."
William Faulkner, *Requiem for a Nun*

Boston Latin School had no entrance exam in 1960. A sixth grade teacher's recommendation sufficed. This all-boys' public school for grades 7 to 12 had been founded in 1635 and was the oldest in the nation. Some teachers joked that Harvard College had been founded the following year to give Latin School's graduates somewhere to go. The first girls would not be admitted until 1972. It offered aspiring kids and their driven families a proven shot at upward mobility. Many of my classmates were first generation Americans, a number from Jewish families fleeing Hitler. The survivors of the Irish potato famine were well represented too. Resolute 12-year-olds from South Asia, Central America, and the Caribbean are more numerous today.

We wore sport coats and neckties every day and were always addressed by our last names only. We were to study Latin for at least four years. The building looked like a red brick box and dated from 1922. Air conditioning was beyond imagination, an exotic luxury for fancy businesses. Indian Summer dictated that in the unmoving air of our classrooms those sport coats would hang and ripen with sweat. Mine was plus-sized to make room for the pads sewn lovingly into the armpits, cutting me an extra husky figure.

As we entered the auditorium that September morning, our eyes were pulled upward to the roll of famous graduates emblazoned in the crown molding. The names of Leonard Bernstein and Joe Kennedy weren't there yet, but Ralph Waldo Emerson and George Santayana testified to the school's academic bonafides. And the nation's founders like Franklin, Hancock, and Adams were well represented. The ceiling was impossibly high, the walls flat white.

The narrow wooden seats seemed a gift from the Puritans, bolted to the aged wooden floor, enforcing discomfort, ensuring alertness. We were mostly strangers to one another, some 500 silent overawed boys filling this severe space. I occupied myself by wiping my wet palms on my thighs.

The headmaster stood on the stage at a battered wooden podium and arched his wildly unkempt white eyebrows as he peered down. He intoned some formal Latin salutation of welcome, paused, then favored us with its translation. He spoke of our great good fortune to be occupying those spartan chairs, then warned that fully half of us would be dismissed by the end of that first year and relegated to our more relaxed neighborhood schools. The eighth grade accepted only 250. The cut would rely purely on our grades.

We had been plucked from every neighborhood in the city and each of us embodied our families' desperate, fanatical dreams. I had been last in every alphabetical line I could remember but now over my shoulder was Aron Zysow. He was no musician but spent his afternoons at Hebrew School. He was thin, dark eyed, serious—did not utter an unnecessary word. His family's exit from Poland was not much discussed. We occupied different bunkers, but I instantly recognized a peer. We became friends as our situation allowed, pulled together by the alphabet.

So—I rode the Cleveland Circle streetcar each day carrying far more than the contents of my bulging briefcase. Those cars were always dense with humanity. Strangers' averted eyes. The smells of last night's dinner and too much perfume, of tobacco embedded deep in heavy coats. I took note of girls in their plaid school skirts, of their pale knees.

I was acutely aware of my mission—to master the Latin declensions, the math proofs, the English syntax, the vocabulary lists. To recognize and recreate the rhythm and architecture of a graceful sentence. The fiddle filled every afternoon. Each evening found me at my tiny desk from dinner till sleep. I took little note of my classmates or of any social life at the school. My duty to history was to succeed in this even now most competitive year of my life, to win a place in the eighth grade. And I did my duty.

Mom and Dad shared their recipe for success on a near daily basis. Whatever *Brown v. Board* might give, some future politician or court would surely withdraw. Whatever came of today's protest or government program, the homework must be my refuge, my preparation for scrutiny more than complete. The world overflowed with enemies, but its contempt would fuel my ascent. I call their words a recipe, but in time they became a catechism. Our world would always be unfair, the treadmill of competition permanent. This trial of selection was natural, almost Darwinian, neither kind nor cruel. I might play on a more level field than they had, but could expect only one chance to succeed, a chance narrower in space and briefer in time than what others enjoyed, must not imagine that the moral arc of any universe would bend toward justice during my brief lifetime.

Our home was narrow too, the ceilings low. My desk lamp was potent, but the other rooms were kept frugally dim. I was often in the subway before the sun found our windows. Mom and Dad had created a bunker—physical, social, psychological. I would come of age in that trench, its walls close at hand. It sheltered and confined, was as secure as their vigilance could make it. The next five years would shuttle me along a well-worn path between school and home via a twilight of packed streetcars and blackened subway tunnels, the world's realities kept imperfectly at bay. Of course, Dad told me about how to behave with the police, outlined the usual strategy of unconditional surrender. But the course and the rhythm of my days segregated me from them—and the "talk" remained theoretical. The risk of expulsion was far less than 50 percent now, though one quarter of poor grades would still mean a talk with the principal. I learned well to read and write—to calculate, to think, to organize—especially to persist. I was making my way in this world.

Boston's segregated schools and the city's violent response to court-ordered busing would soon draw national attention. My place at the Latin School was an oasis, though it felt more like a prison. Racist rhetoric from the school board was blunt. Mom and Dad assured me that the vitriol revealed plenty about the speakers but nothing about me. "Consider the source," they'd endlessly repeat. But their own invisibility belied their confident words. They were, after all, short of money, education, power. Where could they look for equanimity? We three swam in a sea of bigotry, the corrosive message reinforced at every turn, by Church and State, media and custom, a full court press of propaganda.

Each day my briefcase contained the identical bag lunch—peanut butter and jelly sandwich, boxed raisins, and peanut butter crackers. We bought in bulk. A drink came free of charge from the water fountain at the cafeteria's entrance. It tasted faintly of iron. With each use that paper bag would show a new grease spot or tiny tear. I would fold it with delicacy and return it to its assigned nook in my briefcase. Each bag would last several weeks, to the point of disintegration.

Mom and Dad had been forged by the Depression and our family budget aspired to obey the rule of thirds—one third to taxes, one third to savings, one third to spending. I remember Dad handing mom his check on the last Friday of each month. Mom expected to save our way to financial independence, confiding to me that we would succeed "if not in my lifetime, then surely in yours." We were not exactly stricken by poverty but lived as poorer folks than we were. Frugality defined our sense of self—and it was fanatical.

Our clothes were from Filene's Basement, an iconic off-price department store. It came to feel like a second home. Years later, members of its management team helped found a new off-price chain called TJ Maxx. Dressing well was critical compensation for dark skin, but to do it cheaply became an art form. Clothing doubled as body armor against the world's pity. I honed my shopping skills in their husky boy section and struggle even today to reject a serious bargain, despite my overfull closets.

Dad kept his voice tight and his eyes mobile each time we rode the subway, assuring me that the seats next to us would remain empty. He was usually right. We were untouchables, though his gaze was hardly welcoming. He periodically refueled his tank of anger, sometimes by visiting the Brooks Brothers' clothing store close to the Public Gardens in the Back Bay. Once he took me along. He expected to be ignored, and the faux-patrician staff were skilled in not-so-benign neglect. He would not speak—they would not make eye contact. After a few minutes of this dance he would leave, reliably enraged for days. My own feelings now when I enter one of their stores are complex. The regimental ties and gold buttoned blazers have lost their potency, seldom worn but difficult to jettison.

They demanded that my feelings be unknown to the world— and so of course, with practice and time, unknown to me. Repression was a core survival skill, but by now more an impediment, certainly an obstacle to the fullest telling of this story. Mom and Dad quietly insisted that we were on borrowed time in America and had best prepare for its version of Hitler's final solution. As loyal readers of *Jet* magazine, we'd taken careful note of Emmet Till's open coffin. Cash and passports lived under their bed for a quick escape, but I never knew our destination. They were plainly paranoid but would have been crazy not to be.

Corey Road was home to many Holocaust survivors. Their presence cemented our understanding of our own fragile social position but also gave me my first paying job. I earned 25 cents each Friday evening at sundown for flipping on the lights in a nearby home since the Orthodox could do no physical work on the Sabbath. The Silverbergs greeted me warmly each week as their goy Shabbat (sabbath unbeliever). I flicked the switches in one cozy room after another, trailed on all sides by a fussy chatter of Yiddish. The smells of brisket and challah stick with me—also the aroma of many burning candles. I smiled in the knowledge that I was their tool but hoped to feel less foreign as the months passed. I didn't succeed, but I did save every quarter. We admired our Jewish neighbors. Jolly cohesion and law ordered their lives, ritual seemed to armor them against their history. We took close note of their industry, but actually aimed higher.

We aspired magically to become Boston Brahmins, to be Lodges or Saltonstalls. Mom and Dad praised the taciturn restraint they chose to show the world. We imagined them to be fearless, free from the anger that reserved its seat each night at our well-worn dinner table. So, our own feelings were rarely expressed. Public anger could be lethal—Dad compensated at home. Joy was vulgar, like a red shirt or a shouted voice. Fear, though, was permissible. It fueled our days. My decorum at school was beyond reproach, but I counted no friends, only competitors.

I persisted with the fiddle and was enough of a violinist as an eighth grader to enter a new world at the back of the second violin section of the Greater Boston Youth Symphony Orchestra, a serious regional high school ensemble. The skills of the older kids left me awestruck. I had no idea such expertise was possible. I tried to make no obvious blunders and began learning to listen for the orchestra's many voices, to chase the skill of sharing the spotlight, not that it often found us in the second violin section. Weekdays passed in our trench, but Saturday mornings offered a view of the sky. And those rehearsals in 1961 gave me my first exposure to girls, a world away from my furtive peeks into the *Playboy* magazines at the corner drugstore.

My first airplane ride came in May 1962 when the orchestra performed at Carnegie Hall and the White House. President Kennedy extolled the power of the arts on the East Lawn while Jackie sat in the front row in a brilliant yellow dress. I did a credible job with my part in *The Firebird* suite and the *Symphony from the New World*. Lord knows I'd practiced enough.

And in November 1963, as I walked home from the streetcar stop inhaling woodsmoke and autumn air, shuffling through ankle-deep leaves in my too sensible shoes, the Silverbergs' door flew open with a shout of "the president's been shot!" I ran up to our apartment and we glued ourselves to the faraway TV drama as I thought back to the music on the East Lawn and the yellow dress. But life went on and America now had a new president. My routine didn't change. Mom and Dad favored the party of Lincoln in 1960, knowing that Nixon was stronger than Kennedy on civil rights. They hoped for better times under Lyndon Johnson but were acutely aware of his bigoted history in Texas.

I'd been to New York twice before the Carnegie Hall concert. First in 1956 to a night game at Ebbets Field, the Brooklyn Dodgers vs the New York Giants. Dad had driven us 200 miles to see Willie Mays and Jackie Robinson on opposing teams, but my only memory is of an unlit concrete staircase smelling powerfully of old beer and older urine, the pitted stairs then opening by magic onto an endless, impossibly gorgeous green ballfield. And in 1961 we'd gone to a benefit concert at Carnegie Hall for retired musicians' health care. The playing transported me. I still have the program, autographed by violinists David Oistrakh and Nathan Milstein, and remember shaking the stubby right hand of Isaac Stern. The enactment of Medicare in 1965 abruptly shrank the need for these charity events.

We were serious Boston sports fans. In 1956, Dad and I took in the flawless teamwork of the Celtics' Bill Russell and Bob Cousy at Boston Garden. We returned a few weeks later for a deafening hockey game, struggling to see the Bruins' skaters through dense low hanging clouds of cigarette smoke and water vapor. The crowd was fueled by Pabst Blue Ribbon beer, the language from the two guys behind us beyond colorful. Dad jumped up in fury, turned, and yelled at them to shut up. We had to be the only Black folks in the building, but we did survive, and their language did moderate. The beef was over before I had sense to be afraid—and my eight-year-old innocence had been defended. He had run in high school, held the state record at 600 yards. And, though I was chubby and slow, the Latin School track coach recruited me based on that pedigree. Mom rejected the idea out of hand, reminding me that too many Black folks were running and jumping already. No room for jocks in DuBois' talented tenth.

On summer weekends we would sometimes voyage to local beaches. Traffic was always heavy, and a bristling tangle of parental voices invaded every nook of our car's cabin. Dad's hands threatened to strangle the wheel, or at least to bend it, rose toward the roof at moments of particular stress to direct traffic or to express his state of mind. Mom murmured reassurance and I listened in ongoing alarm. His snarls curled against the glass of the windows. No shots were fired but his anger took our oxygen, and I would catch myself holding my breath. Cops, not traffic lights, controlled many intersections outside the city and he was convinced they obstructed him because of his skin. He barked that he was surrounded by idiots, and on arrival at the beach we would fiercely protect our blanket boundaries and keep close watch on our belongings.

But each step from the car recreated me. The sand felt delicious. And there were no violin scales or Latin vocabulary flashcards at City Point or Horseneck Beach. As school pushed me into adulthood, those beaches pulled me back in time. Even now, when I smell and taste the ocean, revel in my buoyancy, watch the clouds drift by and feel the chilly waves rock my body, I'm instantly rejuvenated, once more a kid.

Mr. Sasson now said I merited a better violin and that he had found one for $1,000, made in 1888 in Turin, Italy. It glowed in the afternoon light of my bedroom, its color hovering between scarlet and carmine. It smelled old and foreign, vaguely intimidating. The fingerboard was real ebony, and its cherry pegs were tipped with ivory. The strings were naked steel or catgut wrapped in aluminum and its maker was a man named Enrico Melegari. I was to get a new bow too, not made by machine, but constructed by someone named Schuster. He had burned his name into the wood just above the silver inlay of the frog. The wood came from trees unique to the Pernambuco province of Brazil. This was not a bow to break in anger. Dad recoiled at the price, but our flinty frugality yielded enough money to close the deal.

I, of course, needed no reminders to guard this fiddle well. We had no idea its value could increase over time, but years later they'd name it their second-best investment, outranked only by my education. Away from home it never left my sight. It was first a tool for upward mobility, later a totem of history's power, a reminder that my life wasn't mine. I lived a solitary life—this fiddle was no friend. On many days I would have cheerfully throttled its impossibly smooth, unvarnished maple neck. Sasson insisted I was improving.

STEEP

I was skeptical but began to hope.

Many people think that classical musicians play violins and that fiddles are wooden boxes reserved for lesser music. Not true. Fiddle is a term of endearment, reflecting a bond between player and instrument. Itzhak Perlman describes himself as a fiddler. And Joshua Bell would not imagine his Stradivarius to be anything as remote as a violin. I would discover that bond only decades later.

Trusting that all real musicians could find their way around a piano, Dad somehow wedged one into my bedroom and mom hired Darnell Corbin to be my teacher. Each Saturday afternoon Dad drove me to lessons through a particularly bleak section of Roxbury, reminding me that failure of any kind would consign me to a short life on those hard streets. Performance was routinely and credibly presented as a matter of life and death. Incompetence was, at best, despicable.

He had begun fending for himself at 12 and was in some ways a hard and dangerous man, but the streets had educated him well. He paused once as we stopped at a corner where a kid had been killed a few days earlier in a dispute over 25 cents. As we sat at that red light his eyes scanned his past. He gestured toward a knot of corner kids and quietly cautioned me to avoid folks with nothing to lose, assured me I would know them by their gaze. I never doubted that he spoke from personal experience.

Mr. Corbin was supremely confident. He was a short, stout man who wore many rings, his Caribbean voice shrill and imperious. He enforced the rigors of pianistic technique from his tiny studio over Slade's, his sister's barbecue joint. Dad persevered as taskmaster and loving chauffeur though I am sure he was uneasy with this peculiar man. The smells of the sauces and the bustle of the street rose to envelop us; to distract from the scales and exercises I was parroting without conviction. I would have given a lot for an empty Saturday afternoon, but our family's mission ruled. I sat bolt upright on that piano bench, buried under this mounting avalanche of instruction.

Within half a year they realized that they couldn't manufacture more than 168 hours in any given week for my self-improvement and the piano disappeared. But the catechism did not. My place in the world was precarious, exactly as secure as my most recent performance. Respect I could win. Acceptance, not so much. I credited those messages at my core but was more than relieved to reclaim a few square feet of bedroom and a sliver of time for doing nothing.

1963 found me still in my academic tunnel. I was chugging forward when I confronted a first semester C in Algebra. I had imagined that C meant satisfactory (as the report card indicated), but Mom promptly scheduled a meeting with my teacher, Mr. McCormick. I reported to his room after school and started my homework. The late Autumn sunlight streamed through enormous unshaded western windows that rose to meet the ceiling. I was alone but tried to escape notice, wedged behind a too-small wooden desk bolted to an uneven wooden floor, its black wrought iron legs set too close for my thick thighs, its tilted surface sporting bits of hurried, understated graffiti. The room was hot, the air still. He was magisterial at his own vast, elevated desk, but we didn't speak, hadn't exchanged a word since the year had begun. Mom had left work early and now arrived in a tailored suit and blue cashmere overcoat, courtesy of Filene's basement. She radiated deference. I had never seen her produce such a winning smile.

My gut was knotted, my hands frigid. I didn't know what to expect of this unprecedented meeting but feared the worst. Mr. McCormick was a gray, stooped man. He managed a wan smile as he scanned my papers and assured Mom that merely reaching the ninth grade at this school meant serious overachievement for someone like me, and that I was obviously doing my best. He was on home turf—sure of himself, of me, and of my skin. He was a thin man in need of a smaller suit, his fingertips and lungs too much exposed to too much nicotine for too long. He had been born Irish in a hostile Anglo-Saxon town and would soon retire. As a kid, he'd certainly have seen the signs outside shops and restaurants, "No dogs or Irish allowed." But power had shifted with time, and he could by now credibly imagine himself to be white, that little word with serious weight, with many meanings. On that afternoon he didn't feel any lack of melanin, only an abundance of ease and mastery.

Mom's voice was quiet and docile. She seemed to shrink and he to swell as they spoke. She praised his skill and experience more than once and expressed complete agreement with his judgment. She did ask, though, for copies of the next few weeks' assignments and was effusively grateful to get them. I had no speaking role in this brief and cordial encounter. Smiles and handshakes were exchanged, gratitude repeatedly expressed. I hoisted my briefcase, and we headed for the subway in silence.

The streetcar was slow that afternoon and the whine of the iron wheels on iron rails was disquieting. Seats were plentiful—we were traveling before rush hour. Once home, she said little. No need by now to name our mortal enemy, or to review the existential stakes at play here in this Algebraic arena. She had just delivered her latest master class in guile, her private tutorial in invisibility. Public stagecraft was matched now by intimate fury and deadly zeal for combat. Her breath came quickly. She took grim pleasure in the terrain of this battlefield, reminding me that math gave less scope than English composition for bigotry, that my mission was to deliver bulletproof "letters and numbers." The veins of her neck rose but her voice did not. She hissed that childhood was long past, that Dad would tutor me each night at our kitchen table, that I must certainly become a credit to the race.

The term tough love can't hope to capture her ferocious, glittering eyes and the rage in her whispered voice that November afternoon. More tiger than tiger mom. My fear was as irrelevant as it was intense. I assembled an array of No. 2 Faber pencils and soft oversized pink erasers for the campaign. I might join the "talented tenth" or not. What gift I might have was a mystery, but the coming months of work were easy to foresee. I was drafted that day into the role of child soldier and left more than a few tears on that battered Formica table, but solving quadratic equations came to feel like buttoning my shirt. My academic star rose.

By 1964 I was playing well enough to earn a little money doing local gigs. In April, Jack and Jill, an organization for light skinned graduates of historically Black colleges, hired me to play for their annual reception at the Gardner Museum, which they had rented for the evening. As usual, Dad would drive me to the gig and pretend to restrain his boundless pride while bending every ear in sight. The museum was an imposing Italian villa just around the corner from the Latin School. It sat on what had been a swamp, a fen, and from its entrance I could just see the glow of Fenway Park's lights. Isabella Stewart Gardner, a bohemian Boston Brahmin, had built it in 1903 to house her collection of European art. It was dark and cool even at midday and the paintings seemed to age the surrounding air. She had willed that nothing in the collection could ever be moved, and the poorly ventilated space reinforced that stasis. The art was priceless, although a theft of 13 paintings in 1990 was quantified at several hundred million dollars.

We arrived and headed upstairs, down a long stone-walled corridor lined with faded medieval Belgian tapestries depicting chivalric courtship and combat. The cold of the stone floor crept through the soles of my dress shoes. My hands were already clammy. This venue was a major step up in prestige. And the acoustics would be live—no curtains or carpet, all stone and polished wood. Every note would resound, every error plain as day.

Seated at the entrance to the performance hall was an officer of Jack and Jill, an erect, exquisitely dressed woman, light-skinned to the point of pallor. She greeted me then purred, that as a nonmember, my dad couldn't be admitted. She rose to usher me in—and to face him. They actually knew each other. Roxbury was that small. He hadn't finished college and was fully two shades too dark for Jack and Jill membership in any case. I too was slightly darker than the proverbial paper bag and so also ineligible, but welcome as hired help. My race was perfectly known that night, but ancestry.com would create a new man years later, equal parts Celtic and West African.

I felt Dad stiffen. The moment was wordless. Time stopped.

STEEP

The air closed around us and ceased to move. Violence felt close at hand. Her dismissal of him smacked me, the humiliation so effortless, so perfectly casual and serene, her sense of caste so secure. I heard him hiss, grunt softly, felt his hard right hand lightly shove my left shoulder forward. Time resumed.

The performance space felt like a giant crypt, long and narrow. I'd had my moment of shame but now mined my resources. I had taken to heart those kitchen table admonitions and knew well how to not remember and not feel. So, squaring my narrow 15-year-old shoulders I marched into the hall, smiled graciously, and bowed for the audience. I didn't ask whether I wanted to play this fiddle on this night or whether I wanted to be part of DuBois' talented tenth. I performed much more than a series of notes for Jack and Jill that night, became a trained monkey put through its paces by a decorous cohort of organ grinders. I have no memory of what or how I played but I found Dad where we'd parted, and we drove home in perfect silence in his scrupulously polished 1956 powder blue Buick Lesabre.

I've often wondered how he'd endured that encounter but chose never to ask, to not reopen one of his unnumbered wounds. It could only have been the fiercest love, a love that devoured dignity and erased identity. On that night we weren't so much controlled by history as incarcerated. I can manage a smile today at the irony of such colorist bigotry in that bastion of white privilege. And I know that my sleek audience, seemingly so cohesive and confident, felt as misplaced as I did in that space. But mostly I marvel at the manhood in his restraint, at his resolve to play the long game for his only kid.

Race consumed us, filtered every encounter, colored every thought, walled our world. Anger permeated our minds, ever-present in our silences but instantly ignited by a shared glance between Mom and Dad or a passing reference to his work. To have spared even a little bandwidth for the wider world, to be ambushed by a moment of surprise, would have brought us a sliver of freedom, but our past jailed us.

White privilege is a fashionable term today and quantitative examples abound. They often joked that only with careful planning could a white American manage to fail. But folks born belonging, feeling no need to adapt, surely enjoy such privilege. And they can use its psychological high ground to muster insight or to burnish blissful ignorance. This entitlement is less obvious than the six-fold advantage in median family net worth the Federal Reserve reports for white families, but in its way more potent. This sense of social place prefigures a comfortable, even an affluent life.

We occupied a box canyon of near infinite depth, the air close, the rim a distant mirage. We lived our identity and its politics without public recourse. Our perspective flowed from a ravenous ancestral fear that reliably bloomed into instant, silent rage with each slight, eating our attention, leaving us always more fragile than vindicated. The world's aggressions, micro and otherwise, got far too much of our notice, each collision leaving us more unbalanced. We missed the wide world, packed with its delights and horrors—slippery, astonishing, complex beyond imagination. Our rage was a poor use of energy.

We were impatient and distrustful of politics, but we lionized public figures. The doings of Ralph Bunche and Thurgood Marshall were closely scrutinized, and their blurred images flashing across our 13-inch Magnavox black and white TV provoked silent reverence. Mom and Dad anointed them big people, their tiny images large enough to achieve a sort of divinity, striding simultaneously by some electronic magic into millions of homes. Of course I was to someday join their fraternity, big beyond any dismissive patronage or pity.

We venerated Martin Luther King and donated to the Southern Christian Leadership Council, sometimes more than we could afford. But we resolved also to draw no unwelcome, dangerous attention. We lived as mice, scurrying behind the tapestries of the Ritz. Our money went to Selma while we held our tongues in Brighton. Martin was our hero, had transcended our colored experience, survived the American wilderness, and returned gifting us the grail of his dream. Mom regularly foretold his murder and

STEEP

Memphis proved her right, confirming his heroic bonafides. The rhythm of our lives did not change.

Nelson Mandela was another of our heroes. Mom had (wrongly) predicted his murder too. I traveled with my family to South Africa in midlife, 2003. We would interrupt our older son's year of Fulbright work of exploring the effect of Apartheid's demise on local artists. His younger brother, Chris, was eager to see him. But we were not the only distraction. He was finding time to interview veterans of war—furloughed guerillas, wary spies, aging secret police, hearing what wasn't said, an idealistic American in a very foreign land. He was a gracious host—I recalled Mom's words to him as we made our pilgrimage five miles across Table Bay to reach Robben island, Mandela's prison for 27 years. The wind carried a hint of Antarctica. I was underdressed.

The tour guides were all former political prisoners. Competition for the job was fierce. All were multilingual, all historians sensitive to the many flavors of foreign ignorance. Ours was tall, thin—Zulu, I guessed. He gave us time in Mandela's cell, 7 by 8 feet, a small space for a big person. He then confided as we walked that he was working to remain at ease while seated in the presence of White persons, an old and anxious habit of mind. I wondered at history's power to confine as we stood in this enclosed space, behind the walls of this infamous prison, my own past now more clear, less potent.

A few days later, we left Zack to his interviews and set out north and east for Kruger National Park, a wildlife refuge about the size of Massachusetts. We were to join ten young Scandinavians on a bare-bones safari, sleeping on folding cots, protected from nocturnal predators by a stout electric fence, escorted to porta-potties by well-armed Xhosa youngsters.

Seeing wildlife meant rising at 4:30 and following precisely the commands of our guide Marius, a self-taught Afrikaner savant. His language was Afrikaans, a mix of Dutch and Zulu. I knew his accent only from years of hearing infuriating interviews with Apartheid politicians. I struggled to demolish that memory, struggled to smile. He was not yet 20, rail thin, short, his blue eyes incandescent, his hair nearly white, his teeth impossibly fractured and yellowed for someone so young. Nearly albino. He astonished us by lecturing at length on any animal or natural feature of the landscape we chose to point out, his gaze persistently fixed in the middle distance, attending to us, his charges, only with effort. We were to walk behind him in single file and in complete silence on those early morning adventures, always able to touch the back of the traveler in front of us. Hand signals for stopping and crouching were demonstrated, repeated, stressed. He spoke slowly, his gaze level. "We are prey," he said. "Whatever happens—Do. Not. Run." At our rear walked a silent Black tracker armed with an elephant gun, its barrel big enough to accommodate a golf ball.

Our moment came at a riverbank in tall grass, almost over my head. We had seen many creatures great and small that predawn, but now Marius flashed his signal to crouch. We stopped short as he conferred with our tracker in the low urgent tones of some unknown language. The tracker's gun barrel slowly came up. I heard nothing, saw nothing, but their tension was palpable. 15 feet ahead the grass exploded. A hippo, sounding like an unmuffled pickup, roared past us quicker than any human, breaking the water with astonishing grace. We were now fully alert, and immensely grateful for the expertise of these strangers. The cadence of Afrikaans carried more music than menace that early morning as Marius explained that the ground between a hippo and its water is the most dangerous bit of earth in South Africa. I'd been assured from childhood that political change in this country would require a bloodbath. Not so. I felt for these folks, held them in high regard, knowing that we'd soon leave. I'd gone halfway around the world to amend my past, shelve my future, and confront my present. If only for a terrifying instant.

Imagination was in short supply in 1964. Mom and Dad couldn't see me trusting my life to a teenaged Afrikaner and I couldn't perceive a world without standardized tests. As the 11th grade began our homeroom started taking timed mock SATs. For several years, our predecessors had been debriefed by their teachers immediately after they'd finished those exams, had been pressed to recall as many questions as they could. Now their memories fueled our training, long before commercially produced SAT prep existed. I was making my way in this world by now, running with the fastest crowd in the school, but Mom and Dad still fumed that I'd failed to reach the top of this rarefied heap. My competitors lived with the same imperatives, though, and this pressure cooker was effective. One classmate later headed the Nuclear Regulatory Commission, another was shortlisted for a Nobel prize in Economics. I remember him in tears over his 99% grade on a math quiz.

The word integration was prominent in those years, conjuring some future of unity. But we were disintegrated boys, solitary hunter-gatherers. Geography and culture kept us from becoming friends, but I did learn why our rivals must compel respect. Without them we can't find our limits, can't know whether we've produced our best effort. Our teachers reminded us at least weekly that we were locked into unequal competition for seats at elite colleges with America's most heavily endowed boarding schools, their legacy pitted against our tenacity. And that our predecessors had succeeded without the benefits of new textbooks, a school library, science labs, or athletic fields. The school functioned first as crucible, then incubator, finally as slingshot, propelling its graduates into a richer life. We listened and drilled on.

Our family took religion seriously. Each Sunday I served as an altar boy at two very different churches. Early mornings at All Saints' Episcopal Church in Brookline, where the governor's brother preached and some of Boston's elite worshiped. 11 o'clock at the even more elaborate Saint Bartholomew's Anglican Church in Cambridge, peopled by the local Black West Indian community. I worried constantly about making a false step in those byzantine rites as I swung weighty steel incense containers and moved from one side of the altar to the other at the random commands of an exacting deity. The starch in my vestments abraded my neck and the white robes were short enough to reveal my too-short pants, white socks, and highly-polished orthopedic shoes. The oak pews did not yield to my spine.

Mom would contrast the gleaming Cadillacs in the Cambridge parking lot with the aging Fords in Brookline in her weekly sermonettes on frugality. I grappled at 15 with fine points of doctrinal dispute between Episcopalians and Anglicans and was buried under a mountain of theological dogma but gained some religious literacy in the bargain. And I do remember the weekly prayers in Cambridge for families of lynching victims from places like Alabama or Texas, people mostly unknown beyond the walls of that old sanctuary. I visited St. Bartholomew's in 2019 to find the neighborhood gentrified beyond recognition but the Caribbean congregation hanging on. I reached for my past, but time refused to hold still. Perspective was slippery as I downed a latte at the neighboring Whole Foods.

Mom and Dad saw the obvious hole in my life and moved to fill it by fitting appropriate girlfriends into my schedule. Their network located a girl named Sharon. I had no idea that the Latin School even held a junior prom, but now we were scheduled to go. We all met at her parents' home on the big night, total strangers by any measure. She was brown-skinned and gorgeous, a strapless black dress encasing her body, provocative and graceful all at once. She stole my breath, was an object of instant desire.

But by now I was well aware of my own rank in the caste structure of Black America—an awkward, middling specimen. My cousins had given me impromptu dance lessons at basement parties, and I was credible with the jerk but already too unbending for the slide or the twist. James Brown had nothing to fear from me. And I had nothing amusing to say that night, more fluent in Latin than in banter. Our silences became physically uneasy. I scrutinized my shoes and praised her appearance but had little other repertoire. We danced once—I remember the stiffness of her dress and the silk of her left shoulder. She expertly sized me up as hopelessly alien, culturally deprived.

She headed for the ladies' room and didn't reappear. I stood by its door for too long, shifting my weight in the noise and darkness. Was there a second entrance? Should I burst in, or ask some unknown girl to ask after her? Much too forward. I was slow to accept that night's verdict, too ignorant to be angry. Shame I could manage, though, and crept from the ballroom perfectly put down.

I walked the few blocks to Copley Square, my failure abject but not entirely surprising. The sight of the hulking, gray public library offered reassurance that the world still spun and that I did belong somewhere within it. The building was a refuge, but also a tool, my tack hammer to break into the wider world. I walked across Boylston Street, along the marathon finish line (not yet painted on the asphalt), descended the ancient, eroded granite subway stairs at Copley Square, and caught a streetcar home, incongruous in my shiny polyester tuxedo, though I had thought to remove the boutonniere. The smell of burning iron and the scream of metal wheels on metal tracks felt far away. But my hormones were close, selfish, not easily dismissed. Desperate overscheduling, puritanical parents, and an all-boys' school conspired to pigeonhole young women as objects, objects of fantasy. Managing that myopia would be the work of years.

My self-image perked up just days later. I'd talked to a New York writer a few months before and now my profile interview appeared in *Seventeen*, a glossy young women's fashion magazine. There I was, aspiring fiddler and student, nestled virtually within an array of dazzling models, page after glossy page. They defined American glamor, and their winning smiles helped solace this solitary kid.

1965 pulled me out of my bunker. My SAT results were nearly perfect. Many colleges took note and invited me to apply. We counted coup as we stacked the letters on the hi-fi cabinet. I admired the thickness of the stationery and the exotic watermarks. My star was rising. Amherst and Swarthmore admitted me, and I ached to leave Boston. But the letter from Harvard landed in our mailbox on

Corey Road with decisive weight, validating my parents' sacrifice and exile, really accepting all three of us as a package deal.

I felt no particular thrill. Twenty of my classmates had received the same letter. The guided missile was now in full flight toward its target. I'd met the latest parental demand. The subjugated folks of three centuries were a step closer to vindication. I indeed contained multitudes, had now checked an exclusive box, but would soon meet new obstacles in Harvard Yard. We three had paid the price of the ticket and I got on board. Case closed.

I was in Boston for a meeting almost 50 years later and had been urgently recruited to the Latin School to help judge the annual student oratorical contest known as prize declamation. The speeches by now could be delivered in English (not Latin), but I still protested that I was no judge of rhetorical technique. I was assured that we alumni would cast only honorary votes, that the faculty would have the decisive word. So, I agreed, made my way to the school, and met my four fellow judges. The assembly hall seats hadn't widened since 1966.

To my right was a merry, florid man about my age. Casually dressed, charming. Expensive loafers. He was quintessentially Irish and looked perfectly at home in this weighted space. Conversation flowed easily. As the third speaker finished and we recorded our scores, I ventured a hard truth to this stranger. I whispered my memories of the seventh grade and expressed some envy at his membership in Boston's dominant tribe. I asked how it felt to belong. The fourth speaker began and finished.

He sighed and smiled. "You know, I went to Catholic school through the sixth grade. Mom really wanted me to come here, to public school, to the best place, so she pestered my teacher for a letter of recommendation. On the last day of school, the head nun calls me into her office—I'm thinking I'm up for some kind of prize. She closes the door, pulls out her cane, and starts beating me like crazy. I'm screaming. And she's screaming louder. She yells, 'Do you know why I'm beating you?' She's stopping to breathe each time she hits me. 'Because-you-are-a-traitor-to-the-faith!'

"So," he sighed, "I didn't feel much at home when I got here either." His mouth maintained its winning smile, his whitened teeth perfect, his melancholy eyes peering back into time. History wobbled. I shared this moment of positive regard with my ancestral enemy, shared what the Gospels would have called agape.

As the competition ended and we headed to the school cafeteria for lunch, we walked down a corridor lined with photos of generous alumni. My new neighbor featured prominently, having endowed overseas academic experiences for dozens of his successors.

I'd learned the many ways I could disappoint, but my power to gratify bloomed in the spring of 1966. Late in the afternoon of May 27 our doorbell buzzed. A flat and tired voice floated up to our apartment. "Western Union!" Mom's face hardened. No one we knew got good news by telegram. The skeletal, wheezing courier labored up our steep, narrow staircase. Mom opened the yellow envelope (addressed to me), stared at it for a long moment, then passed it over. The message began "Lady Bird and I are happy to inform you that..." and came from the White House. Her voice pulled my eyes from the text. I was dumbfounded, unable to recognize my own mother. I'd never seen such joy. Strategic victory had interrupted her life's trench warfare. She was ecstatic, literally outside herself, a dancing, singing girl in the body of a 48-year-old woman. Neither of us had any idea what a Presidential Scholar was, but the telegram gave me that designation and invited us all to a White House reception on June 11. We later were told that the Presidential Scholars were picked from the pool of National Merit Scholars by a process which remains a mystery to me.

That same month Mr. Sasson told me I'd been selected to be a soloist with the Boston Pops. Here was validation years in the making, though the Latin School was a concert sponsor and the conductor, Arthur Fiedler, was an alumnus. In any case, I was to play the Bruch G minor Concerto in Symphony Hall and was now officially scared witless. Sasson was clear. Practice until your hands cannot possibly go to the wrong place, then practice lots more.

By then I'd come to understand the value of that practice. The same few notes one hundred times, then one hundred more, seeking a total absence of unintended sound, finding perfect balance and fearless relaxation in left hand and in right, honing a skill living just below conscious control. I knew all this in my head, but my body persisted in trying too hard for too long. The steel and aluminum of the strings cut shallow slices into the fingers of my left hand, slowing my progress. But I pushed on.

And after years of browbeating, Sasson now trusted me with his fiddle. It was made by Giovanni Guadagnini, his loan rather like handing the keys of a Formula One racing car to a student driver. The past had warped our vision. We could have seen extraordinary generosity in his stunning gesture but instead were terrified that I would somehow damage the most valuable object 80 Corey Road had ever seen. Its varnish gleamed golden brown, and it produced enormous sonority and power with minimal effort, as though it harbored a tiny maple microphone. He sold it late in life to buy a palatial Brookline home.

We had a single rehearsal a day before the concert, really just a run-through. The time was mostly for me—the orchestra could play this piece while asleep. I tried to adapt to the astonishing quality of the sound that was surrounding me but had more fun later playing ping pong backstage with the musicians I'd idolized. The ceiling backstage was invisible in the low light. Curtains of infinite length hung from that unseen blackness, fabric covered by a layer of dust as old as the building. Everything but the ping-pong table felt dark and ancient.

I'd often been a soloist, but never for such a large audience. I walked onto the stage that night and noted a bouquet of dozens of flowers behind Mr. Fiedler. For an instant the podium carried the whiff of a funeral parlor. He favored me with an immensely false smile. I remembered where I was, then worked to forget. For decades the world's most famous soloists had stood on these exact planks of wood. This was holy ground. And the hall was hot—I feared that the sweaty fingers of my left hand would stick to the ebony fingerboard, a major problem for shifting.

I was acutely aware of the buzzing of a full house of about 2,500. A squadron of white jacketed waiters delivered drinks and hors d'oeuvres to tables set up on the floor. My own rented white jacket was a good fit for someone else, heavy and already wet in the armpits. But as I looked down, I was reassured by the gleam I'd put on my black shoes. The audience filling the balcony was a blur and the clinking of glasses and plates on the floor atonal, but as Fiedler raised his baton silence fell. My focus narrowed.

My next memory is of hearing backstage that I'd played very well, my anxiety having erased any recollection of the actual event. Sasson was elated. Dad suspected he'd be denied a recording and badgered the radio announcer for a copy of the reel-to-reel tape. The tape was later converted into a cassette, lived for years in my den as a compact disc and is now immortalized in the cloud. As I listen today, I hear a rocky start but a fine recovery, really a credible performance. A job well done. Sasson had often said that I could become a good but not great violinist, and this painful out-of-body experience discouraged thoughts of a musical career. Renown came and passed quickly, but my tribe had been heard. I just wish I could remember something of that night's passage.

In early June we four Presidential Scholars from Massachusetts met in Boston with leading local politicians. House Speaker Tip O'Neill, in his dark oak-paneled office, asked in a booming tenor brogue which of us planned to enter politics. He then filled the awkward silence, speaking rapturously about political combat, valorizing the endless wheel of success and failure, new with each congressional session. He was obviously a natural at this team sport, but all I could think of was Sisyphus and his rock.

The events in D.C. exceeded all expectations. My medal was promptly embedded in Lucite and the photo shaking hands with the president lovingly framed, but the reception in the Rose Garden was the weekend's peak moment. I wish I could have recorded Mom and Dad chatting with people like Thurgood Marshall and Stan Musial, Willie Mays and Earl Warren. Bill Russell's height and cackling laugh hovered over us all. Dad had played against Musial in exhibition games long before he'd reached the major leagues. Now they chatted about players they remembered from the old days. Mom was transfixed as Marshall recounted the stony road from Plessy to Brown.

I was without a frame of reference, mostly struck dumb, repeating a few tired variations on "thank you" in response to the flow of praise from all sides. The food was exotic but delicious. It had not come from a brown paper bag. The grass was perfectly green and the attendants in dress uniform scrupulously attentive. I felt outside myself, a supporting actor in a feature film. Those grainy TV images had come abruptly to life, comfortable in their loose affiliation and in their celebrity. And we three had escaped the box of our history, had trekked from America's margins to its capital, to the epicenter of its culture and its politics. We were at last in the company of those big people, if only as guests. And, on that day, we did belong.

But my most valued artifact from that year didn't come from the president. It was a small, thin aluminum disc, embossed with the image of Benjamin Franklin. It reflected his regard for his school, and the seven Franklin medals recognized the seven best students in each graduating Latin School class. That red brick crucible had shaped me, had readied me for the long haul. Lyndon Johnson wouldn't have recognized the value of that little piece of metal, but my classmates and I knew its price all too well.

-3-
EDUCATED

The euphoria passed quickly. It was time to figure out how to pay Harvard College. National Merit Scholarship money from the Gillette Safety Razor company would help. And the War on Poverty came to the rescue with a work study job in a psychology lab at Mass. General Hospital. I also got work on campus. Both jobs involved excrement—cleaning classmates' bathrooms as a member of the dorm crew and washing out rat cages at the hospital. John Garcia directed the lab and was embroiled in debate with the eminent B.F. Skinner on the question of rodent learning. Skinner maintained that rats' memories were short, measurable in seconds for any information. Garcia had grown up acutely aware that rats in California's Imperial Valley could learn the taste of poison hours after a single sublethal dose, recall it years later, and bequeath that knowledge to their offspring.

Garcia aimed to express his awareness with scientific rigor. My role was to keep the rat cages clear of feces, urine, and dander. The ammoniacal smell singed the membranes of my nose, worse with each afternoon at work. Luckily for me, he was a far better thinker than writer. I gradually made myself useful as his editor and later expanded my job description to become a coauthor on a couple of his papers on olfactory conditioning.

I moved to Cambridge in September 1966, academically overconfident and culturally far out of my depth. I'd live in Harvard Yard like all other freshmen, my dormitory Wigglesworth Hall. The iconic college had grown into a university in 1782 with the founding of its medical school in Boston. And by 1966, it was well established on both sides of the Charles River.

Many of my 1,200 new classmates had inhabited a reliably indulgent world. We traded stories as we moved into the dorms. Summer vacations seemed safe ground. My neighbor said he'd spent two months skiing. I expressed befuddlement until he explained that his family always summered at their mountain home in Chile. Some had made credible, concrete plans to become U.S. senators or Wall Street CEOs, plans realized years later. One was a nationally known concert violinist. They had enjoyed a white privilege completely unavailable to any white person I'd ever known. The word carries a heavy load of meanings—here it stands in for ruling class.

I had come to Cambridge eager to become a new person—to stretch my imagination, to shed my nerd persona. Chasing sophistication, I applied for introductory freshman seminars in creative writing and photography but was soon discouraged to see that one of my fellow applicants had published a fiction piece in *The New Yorker* two weeks before school had started. Other classmates boasted serious photographic portfolios. "Introductory" turned out to be an elastic word in Cambridge. Rejection from those seminars came as no surprise and bent me back toward the natural sciences. Later, the draft lottery would do the same.

I was comically clumsy and invisible at the dim and deafening freshman mixers, a chubby wallflower painfully short of social grace. My clothing didn't quite fit, my language was unpracticed. Many buses from elite women's colleges were parked outside the freshman dining hall for these mixers but their occupants were in search of someone more eligible. I did attract an erudite, introspective girlfriend that autumn. She praised my musicianship and I was thrilled to be the focus of female attention. I took long train rides south from Boston. We exchanged terrible poems and stumbled on carnal knowledge in her dorm room at Bryn Mawr.

The fiddle, that tool for upward mobility, was eating my life. I had long pushed too hard to wring loudness from the old instrument, not trusting its richness and native power. Too much force, too little caress. I did have a musicians' union card and played for a few stage shows in the theater district, but I'd quit practicing. I did still play well enough, though, to play in the pit orchestra for my first opera, a student production of Mozart's *The Marriage of Figaro*. Our conductor, John Adams, became a major composer. And John

Lithgow managed the stage. Richard Gill, a professor of economics, had sung at the Met years before and mined his Rolodex for an amazing cast. These melodies were almost 200 years old but drew full houses each night. Hard to believe we were playing Mozart's first and only draft. His clarity lit up that college dining hall's dead acoustics and the voices raised the hairs on the back of my neck. But the fiddle stayed mostly in its case for the next 35 years.

As a sophomore I decided to join Dudley House, a loose community of commuters, foreign students, and married undergraduates. The decision avoided the expense of the college meal plan and assigned me to live in Harvard Yard for the next three years.

I saved real money by eating at home on many nights and weekends but also narrowed my experience and missed more than a few chances to grow up. Parties, study groups, meaning of life disputes. A residential Harvard house—maybe a community of friends.

I inhaled the liberal arts. I've forgotten much of the natural science I was so anxious to master during those four years but recall points of East Asian history and the development of modern art with delight even today. To see the Chinese Communist Party as the latest in a long dynastic line helps balance the breathlessness of today's breaking news. And as I looked closely from Courbet to Picasso, I finally grasped how Cezanne's apples could weigh so much and how abstract art had come to be. Museum visits morphed from duty to thrill.

The Metropolitan Museum had long been a favorite New York destination and today, October 15, 2011, I'd finally get to visit its Islamic wing. The collection had been hidden in its basement for almost 10 years and the wing's opening had been delayed three times. I bounded up the museum steps two at a time.

The objects were exquisite and their presentation beyond fabulous. The carpets and ceramics pulled me back hundreds of years. The sweep of the calligraphy overwhelmed my ignorance of the Arabic language. I was engulfed by bottomless beauty and infinite intricacy. Allah surely lived somewhere in this geometry and spoke fluently in the language of mathematics. A carpet 30 feet long, all interlocking reds and greens, stilled my busy mind as well as any mantra or Hail Mary. My liberal education had not been wasted. Much of the art I was seeing that day was secular—the human form made its appearance! But the impact was unmistakably spiritual.

Then I remembered where I was—in the cultural capital of our American empire. And thought of some 3,000 citizens dead at the hands of Islamists five miles south and only 10 years previous. I took this collection to be the city's reply and glowed with a moment of intense patriotic pride. As I turned to leave, I noticed a spare figure manning the exit, an absurdly young guard made thinner by his black suit, his eyes in motion, his job taken seriously. His corduroy yarmulke, a sober burgundy paisley, was securely in place, but chocolate brown curls were escaping under its rim. My younger self might not have noticed that headgear. I allowed myself an unthinking moment, chuckled. Baldwin's history was forceful but could wield a flash of deft humor too.

The *New York Times* became a daily indulgence, along with much too much ice cream from Brigham's in Harvard Square. My dorm room was very close to that square—actually a triangular plaza at the intersection of Mass Ave, Brattle Street, and what's now called John F. Kennedy Street. On that plaza sat the encyclopedic Out of Town newspaper stand. I'd jaywalk across Mass. Ave. to reach it, buy the *Times*, then scan the opaque foreign headlines on the pine shelves— dispatches from Tokyo to Cairo, Santiago to Nairobi. That tiny hut was always brimming with smoke, jammed with exotic people and languages, smelling intensely of cigars and newsprint. I couldn't read a word of those papers but felt more hip and sophisticated just being closer to that wider world, brand new every day.

STEEP

The next few steps across Brattle Street brought me to Brigham's, where the butter pecan provided a reliable squirt of dopamine, shaping my adult coronaries and my microbiome. Just like Dad's pancakes, the refined sugar and the praline coated pecans self-medicated, created a refuge from the college's scrutiny. Mostly, the cones just tasted great—sugared, never plain. There was no bad time for ice cream. I would visit for my fix during January blizzards, throwing back my hood and shaking the snow from my boots as I marched in. There was seldom a line on those evenings. The soda jerks would offer a slightly bored greeting. They knew me well. I'd stroll down Mass. Ave, cone in one hand, newspaper under the other arm, duck back into the yard through the massive Dexter gate that accessed the main library's back door, then circle back to my room. I passed through that gate hundreds of times but not until a reunion almost 30 years later did I look up from my shoelaces to read the inscription etched into the arch. "Enter to grow in wisdom." A startling new take on who "big people" might be.

One blistering Saturday two days before sophomore classes began, I spent the morning wandering the aisles of the Coop, the campus bookstore. The smell of those thousands of new textbooks wound into my nose like an exotic perfume. They ran floor to ceiling, wall to wall. The paper, glue, and printer's ink created an intoxicating mix, a fragrance of September possibility, the course offerings seemingly infinite. Was early Coptic poetry real? Could I survive introductory astrophysics? I hit tennis balls all afternoon in Indian summer heat then raced to a dorm party and replaced fluids with far too many Miller High Lifes. I was excited to belong on that night, to seek a world more friendly than I'd been prepared for. The room was unlit but filled with the deafening music of the time, with smoke and shouted voices (mostly male). I belonged a bit too well on that night and a few more. My bedroom spun through the next several hours and my toilet became my base camp. This was a much different intoxication than the Coop had promised, and Miller's High Life had surely been misnamed. I cleaned my bathroom the next day without pay. Garcia the psychologist would have labeled the adventure one trial learning.

Dad took me to a World Series game in October 1967—Boston Red Sox vs St. Louis Cardinals. Having played for the Philadelphia Colored Giants, he was no casual fan. He could typically predict where fielders would position themselves for each batter and what sort of pitch was coming next. Although we were Bostonians, he rooted passionately for the Cardinals because they had hired more Black players. Bob Gibson was his special favorite. We even splurged on hot dogs covered with spicy mustard at two dollars apiece. It was a special day in Fenway Park with a scholar of the game, an abandoned kid fired by incandescent ambition to extraordinary achievement. An American original.

And in November 1968 I used one of my two free student tickets to take him to the Harvard-Yale football game. Yale was heavily favored but the game drew national attention because both teams were undefeated. As we left the Yard and walked down John F. Kennedy Street over the Anderson bridge and across the Charles River toward the stadium, we heard urgent offers for our tickets from sleek alums of both schools. The dollars on offer rose dramatically as we neared the gates, severely tempting us both. I remember refusing $200 per ticket, serious money in those days. I'd often felt alien to the life of the college, but this day was a happy exception. We were lucky to have resisted because the game was a classic, "won" by Harvard 29 to 29.

History shoved me around during the spring of 1969 over the unlikely issue of construction contracts. Mom and Dad had argued hard that I should avoid the antiwar demonstrations that were unraveling the college, insisting that this white man's war wasn't worth risking expulsion and the draft. But those tumultuous times had allowed other local issues to surface. Dad had fumed for years that Harvard's construction contracts went exclusively to white unions. And now Black students planned to draw attention to that policy by occupying University Hall, home to Harvard's administrators.

Confident that my folks would surely support this particular flavor of economic activism, I showed up for the demonstration, although the Student African American Society had consistently found me marginal—a bit too white for real membership—less a problem of skin color than of perspective. I felt the shortest and slowest, last picked for the team. Their sophistication left me feeling somehow excommunicated, stranded on history's wrong side.

The core membership broadcast a single identity, radiated unity. No big tent for them. These pugnacious folks were powerfully charismatic. Their politics were performative but more than real to me in that heady time. They held the world's complexities at bay and owned the truth, heroes and villains fixed in perfect clarity. These were hip creative writers and fluent social scientists paired with righteous, fine girlfriends. I didn't own a dashiki and my fashion statement spoke the language of actuaries. Wonky biochemistry majors lived far from this tribe, the natural sciences hopelessly Eurocentric.

I had been forged to serve the cause, but its demands were changing, the cultural ground of this brave new world shifting under my feet. I was running hard but being left behind—others had found a more forgiving course. The social drivers, the crosscurrents for all of us, were complex. Overcompensation, survivors' guilt, academic animus to rival rising anger in the streets—who knows? The times are always uncertain, but these were very murky days. Adapting to this privileged environment was lonely business. But some of us felt secure enough, for whatever reason, to be provocative. They intended to provoke the college, to draw attention. They succeeded.

I ached to belong to my generation, to that college tribe. The doors of University Hall were unlocked, and we promptly filled its entry without resistance. But as luck would have it, the day after I had joined this, my first direct action, my picture appeared prominently in the *Boston Herald-Traveler*, a popular and sensational tabloid, under a breathless headline trumpeting how a mob of burly and dangerous Negroes had ransacked an effete and decadent ivy league college. My hair was unkempt, my image blown up and blurred, but it was me for sure.

Schadenfreude from family and friends promptly deluged my parents. Pride in their closeted kid had obviously been misplaced, their decade of strategic planning a bust. That pride flipped abruptly to terror and was voiced to me in hard words. "You've wrecked everything we've worked for! Harvard never wanted you anyway! Now they'll kick your sorry behind out and ship it to Vietnam!" Corey Road's walls vibrated. I quivered at my power to wound them, hemmed in by how fused we'd become, shaken by their fear and rage. The college rewrote its contracts a few years later and no one was expelled, but I didn't occupy any more buildings.

Electricity and Magnetism taught an entirely different lesson. Sophomoric hubris had pulled me into a course that was exposing the limits of my cognition. I was seriously intimidated by the professor, Edwin Purcell, a Nobel laureate. I was foundering but of course had been conditioned to struggle alone. After far too long in denial, I faced the humiliation of a visit to his office hours. Six-foot, six inches, stooped, angular, sandy-haired, tweedy, he was the quintessential Harvard Don, occupying much of the space in his tiny, cluttered office. He listened closely to my confusion then astonished me with his patience and clarity. He unfolded his frame, stood, and ambled around his desk to sit face to face with me, our knees nearly touching. He gently pitched his language to my level of understanding as he narrated how relativity had changed physicists' thinking about electricity and magnetism. His voice and his mind felt like a Ferrari engine at idle. He used only as much math as he had to, made certain he'd answered all my questions, encouraged me to return any time I needed to.

His mercy should have upended my bunkered world. I do remember it vividly, after all. But at the time it seemed just a lucky break. My eyes were unprepared for surprise. My past had immunized me against his good turn. I passed the course—and learned that my grasp of the counterintuitives of modern physics was definitely finite.

STEEP

1969 was a tumultuous year for America and its universities. Teach ins, student strikes, grass, beer. Always beer. I lived at the fringe of this action and kept my eye on the ball, became something of an academic, building credentials in neurochemistry and pharmacology. But I didn't pass those years alone. My roommates and I were an unlikely trio of local Dudley House kids saving money on food and making their way. Aron Zysow had been a rival, had ranked one place above me at Latin School and now majored in Classics. He seemed to master a new language each week. He'd come to Cambridge with solid knowledge of Latin and Greek, of course, and had been attentive during his middle school lessons at Hebrew school. Now he added Arabic, Aramaic, and Coptic. His parents spoke little English, so he was obviously fluent in Yiddish and German too. Later in life he taught a course on Islamic law at Harvard Law School and spent a year at the Institute for Advanced Studies at Princeton. He was infallibly reasonable, solitary as an oyster. Innocent of alcohol and dorm shenanigans and, if it's possible, less socially adept than I.

Carl Penndorf was our third. He gave me unwelcome but necessary schooling in our first few days together. I had imagined myself as more informed on matters African than any white kid but was chastened to learn that he'd spent his last high school year in Uganda as an American Field Service student, was knowledgeable in East African history, and fluent in several local languages. He majored in economics and became active in Students for a Democratic Society, a major antiwar movement. Later he joined the CIA (another story).

We spent three years together but knew each other less well than one might expect. Maybe it was the weekends at home. We lived at the center of the college but had few visitors. Aron upended our dining arrangements in 1968 when he converted from conservative to orthodox Judaism, requiring a dedicated sink and a second mini refrigerator. And Carl cost us our common room furniture in May 1969. A phalanx of the National Guard was advancing down Mass. Ave to disperse antiwar protestors occupying

Harvard Square, and our third-floor windows gave us a close look at the confrontation. Though they wore gas masks, we could see that the Guardsmen were kids like us, no doubt grateful not to be in Southeast Asia.

When Carl threw open one of our windows and yelled something unflattering, one looked up and fired a teargas round that by some amazing luck flew straight through that window and into our common room. We were abruptly blind and breathless. Carl reached it in seconds and tossed it out, but our overstuffed Salvation Army couch and chairs were now intolerable, pungent beyond all hope.

Parental visits were complex. Aron's and Carl's parents couldn't be allowed to meet, or so their sons believed. Aron's parents had escaped Poland in 1944 and reached the U.S. after a perilous journey. Carl's Dad had left Europe abruptly too, spirited out of Germany in Operation Paperclip with Werner von Braun and other rocket engineers. They never did meet, but their sons enriched the college and widened my world.

Commencement was to be a peak moment for Mom and Dad, their day of fruition, the definitive proof of belonging that had been so stubbornly elusive. We graduating seniors sat on an array of folding chairs in the stillness of a fragrant June morning at the center of Harvard Yard, just in front of our triumphant families. Mom and Dad were turned out in their best church clothes for this elaborate ceremony and were seated about 20 yards behind me.

But their moment of triumph was suddenly derailed by a crowd of about 20 young rent strikers protesting Harvard's role as slumlord and gentrifier. The complexity of this ancient ceremony made it an easy target—and the college was unprepared for this unprecedented disruption. Commencement was canceled as protestors rushed the dais, forcibly evicting speakers and honorary degree recipients, their bullhorns agitating the morning air. They were well organized, fashionably scruffy, and viscerally provocative. Dad's voice rose easily over the general parental hubbub, offering the protestors extremely specific and unprintable advice involving mostly their mothers and their hygiene. Mom's reminders of the long game were more felt than heard. We wanted to belong—this was not a good moment to upend the American hierarchy. Many of my classmates had boycotted the ceremony entirely. I was there but far from outraged, mildly annoyed but more than ready to move on. And the college did tighten its security. On most days a visitor can enter Harvard Yard through one of about 30 gates. Commencement day now will find about 27 locked, the remaining three manned, open only to ticket holders.

The winter sun sets suddenly in the Colorado mountains. Our family had rented a condo in Snowmass Valley. Now I was walking before dinner, up a narrow road into a neighborhood of rarefied air and exclusive mountain homes. As I climbed, visible houses gave way to dense Aspen groves punctuated by the occasional understated and very unpublic driveway. I rounded a switchback and turned to salute the stars of the eastern sky.

I inhaled the thin air and its woodsmoke, zipped my coat against the north wind. As I turned to descend I sighted a man struggling upward toward me, no more than 50 meters away. He was aged and stooped, gaze downcast, gait uncertain. We were entirely alone, the silence total. We passed without a sign or a word. I looked closely and recognized the steel rimmed glasses of my generation's arch enemy, a member of Harvard's board of overseers decades before, the man who had sentenced so many of my generation to death, the best of the best and brightest now focused entirely on taking his next breath. No security detail.

I opened my mouth, but the mountains' stillness swallowed my anger. I descended a few steps, organized my outrage into eloquence. Although my draft number had been 311 my outrage was fresh. I would unload a piece of my mind on this villain, lay the catastrophe of Vietnam at his feet. I turned, but Robert McNamara was out of sight. This existential threat to my younger self had disappeared. I hustled back uphill to find him gone, vanished into a half-hidden driveway. For an instant I considered pursuit, but my nemesis had melted away like some Wicked Witch of the West, his menace long blown out. My fury faded with the daylight—history's grip relaxed. I worked to reduce my enemies' number, if only by one, and do my troubled mind the favor of clarity, even of forgiveness. Years later, I was moved by the film *The Fog of War*. I stood for a moment struck dumb by the perfect silence and the beauty of the rising moon—and realized I was hungry.

The English word educate flows from the Latin prefix "e," meaning away from, combined with the verb "duco," meaning to lead. Together they convey the process of being led away. And I was led a few steps away from the governance of Corey Road during those four years. My education was underway. The path was by no means painless or direct and its end remained obscure. But I'm grateful now for the deeper understanding of the world and of myself.

I'd also climbed a couple of rungs on the academic ladder despite all the political turbulence and had done some good scientific work. My name had found its way into a few serious journals. I'd spent the previous year in a neurochemistry lab at the Massachusetts General Hospital and with its help had won a Scottish Rite Fellowship. It would let me spend the summer in any lab in the world. The University of Edinburgh sounded exotic but English speaking, yet I was eager to go anywhere. I helped draft a paper there on synaptic chemistry. Though our thinking was muddy and our results unreproducible, I did enjoy the supervised parole from my past and caught my first glimpse of the world in the bargain. I lived in Milnes' Court, a Theology students' dorm a few yards down the Royal Mile from Holyrood Castle, its medieval stone walls two feet thick, its slit-like windows built for defensive archery.

Edinburgh was a city of citizen athletes. Kids were kicking soccer balls on every sidewalk and matrons carrying golf bags strolled the streets. And this was no fashion statement. These ladies were serious players. My lab partners insisted I join them for my first round of golf. I worried I'd embarrass myself. I had never played. The game had been beyond our station in Boston. And this Scottish course was forbidding, more rocks than grass, steep hills and narrow gulches covered in dense knee-high heather. Golf carts would have been useless. There were none in sight. My partners shouted assurances from the hilltop tees and greens that I was doing well in the maze of ravines below. I finished soaking wet and covered with thistles, carding a score of 180, which they said was the maximum allowed. I changed into dry clothes, and we celebrated with a pint, but I haven't played since.

I got no enlightenment that summer from a furtive homeopathic dose of pure LSD lifted from the lab, but my consciousness was altered by the aurora borealis. I chanced to glimpse it as my face froze on a weekend trip to the Isle of Skye. As I headed north from Edinburgh that weekend, I understood less and less of what the locals said. Their tongue had no resemblance to any English I knew. A few weeks later, Eurail pass in hand, I headed for Denmark, Germany, and France. I found a couple of cute girls and sent messages home from the local American Express offices less often than promised.

Inertia and expectations pushed me toward med school. It was safer than southeast Asia, and I was still infatuated with the nervous system. Harvard had admitted me early, and I didn't look hard into the alternatives. I knew every inch and crevice of its neighborhood—Latin School was across the street from the first-year students' dorm. But paying them would be tough. Tuition was $12,000 and although Dad made only $18,000 pre-tax, they offered no scholarship, only a loan at 7% interest. I remember that policy decision each time I open one of their fundraising letters today, though my anger has faded with each passing year. My parents' relentless frugality (and their interest free loans) saved the day. Repayment came about a dozen years later. I barely recall the thick admission packet, this latest step toward some ceremony far in the future when I would be officially recognized as having arrived. I was living in that slippery future, unable to savor even my best moments, running from the past and shrinking my life.

I moved into Vanderbilt Hall, the first-year students' dorm, knowing no one in the class of about 140. We'd been selected to succeed and the school assured us that it would make failure difficult. The building was basic—long straight halls, plain doors and spartan rooms at regular intervals. Its shape was almost pentagonal, with a sunken tennis court at its center. My neighbor across the hall was Tim Russell, a tall, angular MIT grad who hailed from the Bronx. The architecture dictated that we'd see a lot of each other. We shared anxieties and hopes, formed a durable friendship. He invited me to his home for Christmas—a group of twenty played football comfortably on his front lawn and I literally got lost in his house. I hadn't realized that the Bronx contained such a neighborhood and struggled to grasp how so wealthy a family could produce such a driven son. I could barely match his work ethic. He went on to become an internationally-known radiation oncologist.

I imagined myself a psychiatrist. Those I'd known at Mass. General pondered fundamental questions of neuroscience and the human condition. Plus, they dressed well and drove cool cars. Definitely. But Jim Wepsic, a neurosurgery resident and lab mate in 1969, disagreed. He insisted that surgeons weren't necessarily the unthinking mechanics my preclinical science faculty alleged, and that these psychiatrists were literally all talk. He satirized their dialect and rekindled my preference for doing over thinking, that long dormant memory from second grade. I had dinners at his apartment with his wife Karen and their son Eric. Parker Hill was a tough neighborhood then but the medical help he gave his neighbors kept his red Corvette undisturbed.

He sometimes took me on Saturday rounds and one morning hustled me along as he wheeled an old man to the OR, unconscious and unable to move his left limbs. Jim hoped to drain a liquefied collection of old blood, a bleed caused by some trivial, unremembered injury weeks before, a fluid collection expanding slowly within the space between the brain and skull like a dry kitchen sponge grows as it absorbs water from the tap, that growth now increasing pressure within the head, shifting the brain to the point of unconsciousness and imminent death.

He drilled three nickel-sized holes into the right side of the skull. I watched in wonder as what looked like motor oil shot upward out of the skull six inches into the air and the brain slowly rose toward its normal position. The patient woke up immediately in the recovery room and moved his left limbs with reasonable power. He complained bitterly of thirst. This wasn't complex surgery, but these neurosurgeons clearly had the right stuff. They could raise the dead. Still, surgery was so physical—and I was more squeamish about blood than I'd let on.

Preclinical courses like anatomy and pathology filled med school's first two years. Meanwhile, my romance with the nervous system blossomed with our first-year introduction to neuroscience. I was transfixed by David Hubel's lecture on the physiology of vision. Although he'd certainly given this talk many times, the thrill was fresh for me. He walked us through his decades' long quest with no more drama than the subject itself provided. His goal had been to understand how the cat's visual cortex worked. The lab first designed an electrode to measure the electrical activity of those individual visual nerve cells, an electrode strong enough to penetrate a single neuron but fine enough to not destroy it, the work of several years.

Once his lab had built its microelectrodes, it worked to learn what particular visual stimulus would cause a particular neuron to fire. After many failures with colors and shapes, their moment of serendipity arrived when a technician heading home for dinner turned the lab lights off as Hubel was monitoring a neuron at the core of the cat's visual cortex. The neuron fired instantly and reliably as the light switch toggled from on to off.

So, by happy accident they learned that at least one group of this cat's primary visual neurons responded purely to a change from light to dark. He paused. This was breaking news, astonishing basic science. Several more years of mapping revealed multiple families of neurons in a widening anatomic network, increasingly specialized, responding specifically to horizontal or vertical lines, to corners or finally to movement. That this array could work together in milliseconds to register a stealthy mouse was miraculous.

H. Richard Tyler, a skilled neurologist and gifted showman, presented us a case of Wernicke-Korsakoff syndrome, in which no recent memories can be retained. Its two most common causes are intoxication with carbon monoxide or alcohol, injuring a tiny structure deep in the temporal lobe. His patient that day looked like a silver-haired banker. Dr. Tyler greeted him, chatted a bit, then excused himself. When he returned a minute or two later to resume their conversation his patient was witty and eloquent, but politely insisted they'd never met. He repeated the encounter several times with minor variations to fix it in our long-term memory. And he succeeded, at least for me.

Med school's third year took us out of the classroom and into a series of one-month clinical rotations in the teaching hospitals. Knowing I didn't want to be a surgeon, I chose to slog through general surgery first. I expected a poor grade because I'd have no idea what I was doing but knew that the experience would make me more skilled for my later, more consequential psych rotation. I trusted that third year students didn't get near a scalpel, and that the surgical rotation was mindless and grueling, work weeks alternating between 72 and 144 hours, more hazing than education. Corey Road had governed my younger days but at least the sleep of those nights had been undisturbed. I also knew that the surgical hierarchy in a teaching hospital was quasi-military and carried a distinct whiff of misogyny.

As it turned out, I knew nothing. The month flew by, my attention to the task at hand entirely undivided. Success and failure were clear in real time. The illnesses and their treatments were not theoretical. I was at the bottom of a hierarchy but felt no malice. For once I felt more real, more necessary than superfluous. The White Building at Mass. General was short of orderlies and phlebotomists. Nurses were scarce. So, if we med students didn't transport patients, change bedpans, draw blood, and run specimens (with correct requisitions in triplicate) to the lab, our surgical team simply couldn't function. I reported 24 hours of my patients' data to my intern at 5 a.m. each morning so that he could relay an edited version to the full team on rounds at 6 and cases could start at 8.

The pockets of my too short, too tight white coat overflowed with pens, requisitions, tourniquets, stethoscope, and penlight, not to mention my "peripheral brain"—a primer for surgical interns. I didn't treat that little book as well as I'd cared for my Latin School lunch bag, and it frayed quickly. I did learn to draw blood, leaving in my wake a trail of multiply-punctured, quietly irate patients. But many of them understood the larger transaction; they received care from world renowned physicians surrounded by a flock of less expert interns, residents, and students. I have immense gratitude for those irritated folks. My future patients would gain from their predecessors' discomfort.

As I learned to recognize serious illness and manage fluids, I was rewarded with permission to close simple wounds and start central IV lines. We were seldom tempted to overdiagnose or overtreat our patients since all the attendant work would fall to us. My grade was a major surprise. Abruptly, I was more of a physician.

Rotations came and went, but fascination with the nervous system persisted. I had finished the required clinical clerkships by the end of the third year and chose to spend my last year with small rodents.

My advisor would be Verne Caviness, a young neurologist I'd met three years before when he'd been a teaching assistant in our Introduction to Neuroscience course. His skills had been memorable. I'd worked in several labs but hadn't done truly independent work and I felt he'd have a lot to teach me. He focused on developmental neuroanatomy in his bargain-basement lab a few miles from Boston at the Fernald State School for the Retarded in Waltham. The lab's immodest goal was to understand how the mammalian cortex came to be. The cortex is the brain's covering, its fresh coat of paint, its most superficial structure, added to our mammalian nervous system only about 200 million years ago. It contains billions of neurons in a six layered array, and though it averages only about a centimeter in thickness in humans, it manifests all our conscious functions— sensory, motor, and intellectual. Cause for wonder.

But his first lesson in the autumn of 1973 was more elementary than wonderful. Which scientific questions are good, and which are not? His answer was that good questions are those we had tools to answer and whose answers would yield more good questions. Those answers in turn would carry the intrinsic value of basic science, even if clinically useless in 1973.

Our lab had three tools. First, the light microscope, developed in about 1590 and familiar to every student of high school biology. Second, stains—specific chemicals absorbed by neurons and visible microscopically. And third, rodents. Populations of normal baby mice and strains of evocatively-named mutants like Jimpy, Weaver, Staggerer—and Reeler. These damaged critters were tiny, their white fur soft beyond description, their restless eyes perfectly scarlet. The disturbed circuitry of their brains undermined balance and coordination enough to make feeding and mating difficult. Reeler's individual neurons looked normal under the microscope, but they weren't organized in the normal-six layered array. They seemed randomly placed, sending these mice reeling through their shortened lives.

Neurons have three parts: a cell body with genetic information and metabolic machinery, many short dendrites to receive electrical signals, and a single longer axon to transmit them. Axons communicate with their target dendrites in other neurons across tiny spaces called synapses. Silver stains for axons, brilliant black under the microscope, had been available for many years, but the world of neuroanatomy was energized that year by the discovery of a new enzymatic stain, a peroxidase that was absorbed by axons and transported *back* to their cell bodies. Its rosy-pink color was hard to miss. How anyone had thought to look for it in horseradishes I never understood, but horseradish peroxidase was now our newest tool, allowing us now to locate a very few cell bodies in an otherwise impenetrable thicket of millions. Now we could map both the comings and goings of those neurons we had managed to stain. My roommates, meanwhile, were delivering babies, reducing fractures, unraveling electrocardiograms. My mice and I lived beyond the pale of clinical training, strangers to their shop talk.

But—we had our good questions. Was Reeler's cortical disorganization truly random? Did it result from an error in migration of neurons in the maturing brain? And how did that disorganization affect how Reeler's neurons communicate (or synapse) with each other?

Good questions, yes, but Verne's second lesson turned to the payment of dues. No one was eligible even to raise these questions without a fund of technical and scholastic knowledge. The technical knowledge came from the lab itself. Reproducible technique was the coin of our realm, at the core of what science was. Operating consistently on these tiny rodents, later guillotining them without brain injury, gently removing the brains, freezing them promptly in dry ice, synthesizing stains, creating reproducible paper-thin brain slices with our antique microtome, applying the stains, and finally fixing the unwrinkled slices to glass slides. Scholastic knowledge came from the library, sifting through decades of neuroanatomic research in seldom-referenced, antique European journals—unraveling the arcane taxonomic disputes, the bold false starts, the glacial retreat of ignorance.

I doubted I'd become eligible in a single year to ask our questions but did manage to make the journey my destination. I came to enjoy that quotidian routine at the heart of basic science: the passion for reproducibility, for consistency, the drive to eliminate variables, the relentless skepticism. And I came to believe that if I stained the same spot in the same way at the right time in enough mice, I might get a peek into their cortical architecture.

Making that belief real was the work of nine months. Each day I'd find some new way to fail, and each day Verne would respond with his deft mix of severity and support. He and his accent very much hailed from the hills of North Carolina and rumors within the department whispered that his origins would retard academic promotion. Instead, he became a beloved and world-renowned professor of pediatric neurology. I've not had a better teacher, before or since. He taught me to respect my predecessors, to follow protocols, to mistrust my own brilliant insights. That is, to adopt a modest, antique conservatism that resonates far beyond the laboratory.

The result arrived in March. But first, the roadmap. The mouse cortex contains six layers of neurons. And it's thin, averaging a bit less than one millimeter. It covers the deeper white matter of all the lobes of the brain like the peel covers an orange. All its neurons arise as stem cells from a central embryonic tube, the deepest layer of cells only a few days after birth, each subsequent layer migrating from that tube past its predecessors, pushing to reach its final, more superficial position, creating billions of synaptic connections on its journey. For context, consider that our human brain at the same point in maturation is generating about 250,000 new neurons per minute.

Picture the mouse cortex as a cotton ball cap lined with fur, its bill at the front and the snap in back. The normal cortex would look—well, normal, the bill and snap front and back. Reeler's bill and snap were in normal position too. But large patches of fur would somehow appear at random on its cap's cotton *surface*. Why? How to unravel this microscopic chaos was our good question.

That March morning, I was looking at a slide of Reeler axons entering the deepest cortex from the opposite hemisphere. The black-stained fibers were ascending from the sixth layer toward the first just as in the normal mice. But then I saw one, then another, then a third execute an abrupt 180-degree turn, diving back down toward the deepest sixth layer. As I focused the microscope up and down, more and more came into view. I'd been ambushed by the sublime.

No one had ever seen this. I was the first. I knew that because I knew the literature, because I had remembered enough German from

Latin School to have paid my dues to those dusty, disintegrating journals.

I looked, looked again, stood, walked away from the microscope, breathed, peered out the lab's tiny, smudged basement window, cautiously returned to the bench and looked once more to assure myself that those axons hadn't vanished. I called Verne over. He agreed. This was real. And it was important. We realized at that moment that these axons weren't growing toward a fixed location in the cortex but were somehow drawn downward back toward their target dendrites and cell bodies. We surmised on the spot that Reeler's cortex wasn't thrown together randomly but actually built *inside out*. And now we could ask our next good question, could ask why it was inside out, maybe because each new wave of migrating neurons in those juvenile mice was somehow blocked by its predecessors. We had one new fact about how the mammalian brain is built. We had our answer. And more good questions.

The memory of that morning is perfectly clear after 50 years. I had tasted the rigor of basic science and could now see it as more a way of thinking than a technology or a machine. As an eagerness to make one mistake after another, each a bit closer to a truth. I could also recognize sloppy thinking and lazy work. I'd bring a discerning eye for junk science to every academic article and breathless breakthrough I'd ever see.

I had glimpsed something like a cloudless night sky through the lenses of my Olympus microscope. It was a transcendent moment, literally a moment brimming with wonder. We had been diligent and skillful. And so, we had been prepared for that stroke of luck that let us untangle a bit of elegant neurologic design. I'd veered from Corey Road's assigned trajectory, but my year in the company of those mutant mice had been well spent.

Mom and Dad, meanwhile, had returned to the suburbs, this time to a larger ranch house in Framingham, a western suburb of Boston. It sat on a corner lot and Mom assured me that the extra square footage carried unquestioned prestige. I spent Saturday mornings there when I could, relishing Dad's pancake breakfasts and dreading the mowing that followed. More space to own meant more lawn for me to mow. I seriously questioned the value of that corner lot as I pushed our ancient mower through stifling humidity, lurching back into the house two hours later a wheezing soaking mess. Surely, I deserved better. Where was the leisure for this almost-physician, this credit to the race? Certainly not on that suburban lawn, yoked to a mower built of oak and iron. Many of us imagine that our work has a beginning and an end. The grass knew better.

Med school would end in 1974, and a career decision loomed. Internship and residency. My education was moving along but my past still blurred the present. My classmates were a rare breed, chosen carefully to be leaders in medicine. I learned too little of them and I regret the myopia. I was pulled by the nervous system and by surgery, so of course I would shoot for the moon, aspire to become a top gun, a neurosurgeon. As with med school, the path seemed determined, but by whom, or what? I'm amazed now about how little I knew about the nuts and bolts of neurosurgical life when I embarked on it, but a stew of intellectual curiosity, altruism, and blind ambition propelled me. Professional training would become my next layer of body armor as I chased the world's unqualified respect. Goodbye forever to pity, ridicule, contempt. The drive to be big, the aspiration to be recognized felt endless. And indeed it was, the armor ever thicker but never perfectly trustworthy.

I was very much a Boston guy, and my residency advisor doubted that competent neurosurgical training could actually occur beyond the Harvard teaching hospitals. But my urge to move, to change the script if only a little, hadn't weakened since 1966. I interviewed at Columbia in New York and McGill in Montreal. I learned there that Doctor Penfield Avenue is the only street in the world named after a neurosurgeon. And in November 1973 I flew to San Francisco with Tim Russell. We would interview for internships at UCSF, he for internal medicine and I for neurosurgery. We'd crash with our former roommate, who worked as a dental hygienist and blackjack dealer to afford her apartment in Pacific Heights.

We left Boston in a freezing drizzle and landed in San Francisco on a gorgeous afternoon. The smell of eucalyptus enveloped me as I got out of the cab and remains among my strongest memories of the city. The view from Alta Plaza, her neighborhood park, captured my breath and my heart.

I rode a jammed Muni bus south through Haight Ashbury to UCSF early the next morning for a full day of interviews, the last with Charles Wilson, the chair of the Department of Neurosurgery. He was part Cherokee, short, rail thin. His Missouri twang rattled into my head, and a severe buzz cut dramatized his prominent ears. After about 30 minutes he bent the rules of the residency matching program to offer me a job on the spot, promising to rank me number one if I'd do the same for UCSF. The department offered good clinical experience in those days but didn't support much research. He went on to assure me that it would soon become the finest training program in the world—and managed to make that astonishing idea sound perfectly reasonable. I felt recognized, my years of persistence validated. I dreamed that I could be a new man in this new place, could exit Corey Road's bunker, could find freedom and grow up.

Med school commencement came in June 1974 without the drama of rent strikers, a quiet echo of the events of four years before—165 new doctors reciting an abridged version of the Hippocratic oath. We enjoyed good food and drink under the cover of several acres of white canvas tents. A litany of forgettable speeches followed. I gave a short one myself. Mom and Dad had a moment of pride tempered by the knowledge that their son would soon be gone, launched into six more years of preparation. My mind had left Boston, though my body attended the ceremony.

-4-
THE BETTER ANGEL

I fledged at 25. Mom and Dad waved goodbye at Logan airport, and I flew to the city by the bay. I tried to inhale everything about this astonishing place in the week I had before the ordeal of internship began. Those days were endless and glorious. The smell of the Pacific wound into my nostrils each morning. I could set my watch by the afternoon fog. The air was chilly but perfect. I tested my competence by renting an apartment and furnishing it. The budget was tight, but bargains were everywhere. Used furniture from the Mission, art prints from the Castro, kitchen equipment from the Sunset.

It was all so new—the Embarcadero, Union Square, North Beach, Chinatown. On and on. The scent of eucalyptus defined Golden Gate Park. The roar of the ocean was just audible through my open window in the early hours of the morning. So now of course I wanted to have my cake and eat it, to become a neurosurgeon while enjoying life as a tourist. But no. I had had my liberal education. Next came training.

Surgical internship began June 20, 1974, with a month at the Fort Miley VA hospital, tucked into the northwest corner of the city. Its back door opened out onto the Golden Gate Bridge and the Pacific Ocean, a view I rarely stopped to enjoy. The hours were as advertised. Every other night and every other weekend on call in the hospital. We interns moved each month through rotations like obstetrics, general surgery, or ER in UCSF's three teaching hospitals (VA, Moffitt, and San Francisco General). Our short week worked us Tuesday and Thursday nights (but of course 12 hours on all the weekdays too) and came to 72 hours. On the long week we covered Monday and Wednesday nights, as well as the entire weekend—

Friday morning till Monday evening—and clocked in at about 144 hours of work, or immediate readiness for it.

Today we see those working conditions as crushing or dangerous or both. They've long since been modified. But full immersion into serious illness did compel us to live with it, to recognize it by reflex, to sort sick from well in a heartbeat. Sound decisions became as habitual as breathing, day or night, alert or exhausted.

My new bunker was tucked into an exquisite urban landscape. Each month I had two Saturdays and two Sundays off. One Saturday, after addressing a pile of laundry 12 days' deep, I strolled through the Marina and was amazed to see so many young healthy people out and about, living normal lives. These folks were upright and taking nourishment, wore stylish clothes, and were without catheters or drains. Some were beautiful. Their Saturdays seemed to be rolling easy.

I hung with a different crowd. I hadn't yet graduated to the status of first-year resident, but I did reside at the hospital most days and nights, my companions the halt and the lame, the sick and the dying. I took on some exotic knowledge during that year but on a more practical note I became expert at starting IV's. My best teachers were the heroin addicts admitted to San Francisco General Hospital (SFGH) for treatment of abscessed limbs or infected heart valves. Their knowledge of venous anatomy was encyclopedic, and I was grateful to learn.

Current events overran my bunker in the spring of 1975. I was on the general surgery service at SFGH, my task to keep our patients alive from one hour to the next and to do the occasional small operation. A San Quentin inmate had been admitted the previous day with peritonitis, a serious inflammation of the membranes enclosing the abdominal organs. He had complained of abdominal pain for days, but solitary confinement had delayed his diagnosis of a ruptured appendix, complicating a common illness. Membership in the Black Panther Party had not expedited his care.

He was at SFGH because San Quentin, and Marin County, had

STEEP

no jail ward. Ours was within the building but a full five-minute walk from all the other patients. My junior resident, one rank above me, had done the appendectomy 12 hours earlier. I was to include this new patient on my pre-rounds that next morning. To check his urine output and IV fluid intake, his incision, his lab work, pain status and meds, to make necessary changes and report his status to the team at about 7 a.m. Because he was so distant from our other patients I decided to see him first, at about 4:30.

His name was Fleeta Drumgo. He was only two years older than me but had lived a different life. He'd been convicted of burglary in 1967 and was serving time in San Quentin when he was accused in 1971 of being part of an attempted escape in which three guards and three inmates were killed. His radical politics made him an easy target. The trial had riveted the nation, and his acquittal did nothing to dampen the existential white fear the Panthers provoked. Like many middle-class Black folk, I was uneasy with their apocalyptic rhetoric but had to admire their near suicidal courage and honesty. He was ultimately released in 1976, but in 1975 he had belly pain and found his way to our service. He would be closely guarded.

I was aware of the politics but would focus tightly that early morning on Fleeta's clinical situation. I'd often rounded in the jail ward and was in my usual hurry as I reached its entry checkpoint. I showed my badge and was buzzed through the steel door by a familiar, very bored San Francisco cop. We nodded in mutual recognition. I hustled down the ward's long central hall, passing the shorter corridors coming off at regular intervals to the left and right. The walls and floor were bare. Fluorescent ceiling bulbs banished every shadow.

I turned right to head for Fleeta's room and instantly registered an altered landscape, a foreign face—a man younger than me sitting on a steel chair next to my patient's door. He was chalk-white, fit, dressed in the uniform of some unknown security force. He wore a Kevlar vest and balanced an M-16 assault rifle across his thighs. He was also asleep. I had made no effort to be quiet as I turned, and as I moved forward, his eyes popped open. He rolled off his chair to a prone position and trained the muzzle of his rifle on my chest before I could take another step. We were about four yards apart. His breathing was ragged, and I hovered at the brink of incontinence, my shoes nailed to the floor. I did not move or breathe, had no time to regret my 'fro.

After a brief eternity, he recognized me as more white-coated Good Humor man than urban guerilla. He coughed softly and resumed his seat with a hint of formality, waved his rifle to guide me into Fleeta's room as though nothing unusual had occurred. We did not speak. Our eyes met as I passed his chair, and I tried to piece together some semblance of bedside manner as I greeted my patient, asking about pain control and listening for bowel sounds. I asked that he alert his nurse when he first passed gas, our signal that he could begin to eat. Our doctor-patient relationship was constrained by my overturned state of mind and by his four-point leather restraints, but he did manage a tiny smile at the thought of food.

Later that day I sat at a nurses' station between admissions and tried to recover myself, wondering how the press would have covered my death. Of course, I would have received brilliant trauma care five minutes down that long hall, but would certainly have succumbed to a wound from that weapon at such close range— Pillsbury Doughboy perishes in case of mistaken identity? Colleagues mourn? Attention would have migrated promptly to more urgent concerns. I had imagined I was training in a bounded world, but this random encounter exploded my narrative and nearly put an end to me. Fantasies of past and future had been momentarily erased.

I moved more slowly and made more noise the next day. And Fleeta had a new guard. I rotated off the service a few days later. He recovered well and finished his burglary sentence the next year but was shot dead in Oakland in 1979. No motive was established, and his two assailants were never found. Internship continued.

Neurosurgery residency began the following July. Two residents began this five-year journey each year. I was paired with Isabelle Richmond, recently an assistant professor of neuroanatomy at Duke and the program's first woman. One of that year's chief residents, Bob Spetzler, went on to become the world's leading neurovascular surgeon. I had my own credentials of course, but sometimes wondered how I had landed in this group of 10, and how exactly I'd be revealed as an impostor. Several of us seemed to take to this training with joy, as though they'd been born to this stony path. I was moved as much by duty to history and envied their delight. I feared that driver might not be enough, might fail to move me through the darkest moments ahead.

Six-month rotations again were spread over the three hospitals. The faculty's goal was to gradually increase our level of authority and responsibility in tandem, but because of a scheduling shuffle I found myself the chief resident at SFGH in July 1976—a year too soon. The rotation had long functioned as a trial by fire, a big step up in responsibility. All major trauma cases in San Francisco County came there by local ordinance. The resident lived in the building for that half year aside from four weekend days off each month when a faculty consultant provided relief. I began each day fearing that I'd be called to the OR for endless hours, so I girded myself by eating all the free carbs the hospital cafeteria could offer, day and night. The doughnuts kept the trials of surgical performance briefly at bay and I graduated from large scrubs to XL.

My first month held the usual mix of elective cases, consultations, and trauma. In early August I met my most memorable Jane Doe. She came from the Barrio surrounding the hospital, had the face of an Andean princess, an elfin body lost on the full-sized gurney. She offered no date of birth. I guessed her to be twelve. A truck had thrown her from her bike only a few minutes before, leaving her unconscious but nearly unmarked. She made no response to my shouted voice and grunted as she inhaled, arching off the gurney to my lightest touch, all her weight borne by her heels, her fists, and the back of her head, a deadly posture known as decerebrate rigidity. Her pupils were unequal, left larger than right, and made no reaction to my penlight. Ten seconds of neurologic exam showed that her brainstem was under serious pressure, probably from the left. Death was close at hand.

The ER's preparations for emergency surgery were well-oiled. We were on our way to the OR in less than five minutes—clothing sheared away, lines placed, blood and urine to the lab, screening X rays of the chest and neck done—and read by me. I shaved her hair and stuffed some into a plastic bag either as her property or as an aid to her mortician, the rest falling to the floor. No family. No signed consent. Time for me to step up.

I gave myself permission to explore the space between her left brain and skull, hoping to find and remove a large blood clot. If no clot was found, her problem would be one of major swelling within the brain and her death even more likely. A CT scan would have allowed us to avoid this surgery, but San Francisco's designated trauma hospital was the last in the city to get funding for a scanner, in 1978.

Surgery began with three left-sided nickel sized holes into the skull, drilled with a hand powered spherical steel burr at the locations most likely to harbor a clot. We'd already begun the usual treatments for brain swelling in the ER: aggressive hyperventilation and an IV blast of the diuretic mannitol. The hole just in front of the left ear yielded a spurt of maroon clot, enough to justify a full craniotomy. I'd opened many heads in my first year and now moved with ferocious speed to make a scalp incision about 12 inches long in the shape of a giant question mark. My hand-powered Gigli saw, a thick steel wire lined with razor teeth, slithered into the tiny space below the skull. I attached handles to each end of the saw, allowing me to pull it back and forth, sawing through the bone and connecting the three holes. A section of skull the size of a dessert plate lifted away easily within a few seconds. Beneath the skull was the leathery membrane called the dura mater. It was rock hard, reflecting a deadly increase in pressure below. I opened it to reveal a clot immediately under my temporal burr hole as I'd expected, but also a wide expanse of frontal and temporal cortex more purple and angry than anything I'd ever seen. The worst news. Serious swelling. No big clot to remove.

Time to close—to replace the plate of bone and close the wound—and to do what was possible to treat this swelling with medicines and hyperventilation. But in the minute I'd spent irrigating away bone dust and controlling small dural bleeders the brain had risen over the edge of the fixed bone, making replacement of the bone plate impossible. Cortical bleeders now appeared more quickly than I could control them. This was malignant cerebral edema, a problem of academic interest for me until that moment. The cortex began to rupture at several points and within five minutes had risen level with the scalp. My cotton gown was heavy with sweat, and I was desperate to disappear from this operating room, but also compelled to somehow close the wound I'd created.

The anesthesia resident reported bright red blood from the tubes in the windpipe and the bladder. He said that we might be dealing with disseminated intravascular coagulation, a newly reported condition neither of us had ever seen, in which patients bled uncontrollably after they had exhausted their native clotting mechanisms. The recommended treatment with the blood thinner heparin seemed beside the point as her blood pressure sank and urine output ceased.

Bits of semiliquid brain and clot began to slide down the surgical drapes onto my gown as I stood at close quarters with this catastrophe, my belly pressed against those drapes, brilliant lights hovering over each shoulder. Jane's blood mixed with that of unknown donors to turn my Kelly-green OR clogs a mottled purple and paste my scrub pants to my legs. Closing the scalp now would require amputation of lots more of this mushrooming dead tissue. As her blood pressure dropped her bleeding inevitably slowed, and I wondered for an instant where she'd been going on her bike, wondering who might have been expecting her.

I called for heavy nylon suture and, as the scrub nurse and I leaned hard onto the swollen scalp flap, produced an ugly one layer running closure with my free hand, like a novice tailor might have thrown together a hem. I spun three extra layers of gauze around the head to retard the ooze and temper her family's horror. Her blood pressure fell to zero as we reached the recovery room. OR time was one hour and ten minutes.

It was my first intimate encounter with violent death, death at my own hands. And though we were strangers in life, Jane Doe became the first of a community of ghosts to live inside my head. My blue scrub shirt clung to my chest, and I shivered as I scrutinized the tiles of the recovery room floor, resolved not to vomit before I could finish dictating my operative note.

Mercifully, my memory of the next few hours has more than its share of holes. I surely changed into fresh scrubs to meet with the family and the police. I am sure that voices were raised in pain and tears were shed in that tiny conference room. But I'm also sure that I made rounds that evening and operated the next morning. I'm sure all this happened but have no memory of any of it. Those hours found me diminished and alone. I owned this catastrophe utterly, had failed my family's prime directive of competence. I worked to see through my tears. But having not known Jane alive, I would soon struggle to mourn her. My beeper continued to chirp, the parade of mortal maladies went on, and the city's exquisite beauty was untroubled by Jane's demise.

I presented her case to our weekly death and complications rounds a few days later and, in what passed for PTSD counseling, heard from my senior professors in the most matter-of-fact tones that my experience had been far more common in the days before osmotic diuretics and mechanical ventilators, that the lesson was to recognize this particular face of death more quickly. All agreed that she was past help from the moment her head had hit the pavement of Valencia Street. So now I was abruptly older, harder, more efficient under duress, a bit more of a surgeon. Experienced in ways future patients might rather not know.

SFGH brought trials but also redemption in the person of Harold Rosegay, my faculty consultant. He was a fine violinist and a rabid boxing fan. I remember him teaching me a bit of Sugar Ray Robinson's footwork one morning as we stood at the scrub sink.

Years later we would play string quartets upstairs at his home in Sea Cliff. During those visits I tried to sit with my back to the glass north wall of his study to avoid the distraction of the Golden Gate Bridge, which seemed to originate from that very room. He'd been the senior American neurosurgeon in Vietnam, returning with an endless variety of jokes and a level eye for triage.

I called him in a panic on the night of the Golden Dragon Massacre. The Joe Boys were hunting their rivals, the Wah Ching. They exchanged many rounds but managed to shoot only patrons of that Chinatown restaurant, killing five and wounding 11. A friend raised in Chinatown later told me these wannabe gangsters probably had never fired a weapon before that night. Harold separated the quick from the dead at a glance and showed me the meaning of speed in the OR.

The rotation was, after all, a trial by fire. It came close to the midpoint of the five-year program and told the faculty a lot about a resident—temperament, skill, judgment. So, I seldom called Harold. But he magically appeared when I needed him most and showed amazing patience with my ignorance. Mostly he kept me from doing serious harm. As my so-called assistant, his role was to keep our surgical field clear, his only tools a saline irrigating syringe and a variety of small steel suckers. As the principal surgeon I wielded the dangerous instruments—the electrocautery, the dissectors, and the fancy micro scissors. I tended to confuse expertise with complexity, but he knew that the simplest approach is usually the safest. Every quick detour meant more bleeding, more time, more hazard. And, of course, surgery requires a field clear of blood and smoke, meaning that the humble sucker actually allows the surgeon to see, and so directs the path of the operation.

I remember moments when his sucker suctioned, retracted, dissected, palpated—was a small tool with many talents. Doing neurosurgery is difficult, but teaching the skill is far more trying, demanding rare wisdom and generosity. Harold was surely wise and generous, but selfless is the adjective that best captures the man.

He demonstrated the special mix of mercy and violence that

defines our calling one day in October. I was asked by the gynecology resident to see a woman terminally ill with metastatic cancer of the uterus. Her problem was intractable, horrific pain, his question what we might do to relieve it. She was bedridden, every bone in her pelvis and lower spine eaten by tumor. Her vital organs were riddled, the smell of her decaying body apparent well up the hall from her room. Her narcotics weren't relieving her pain yet left her too impaired to communicate with her family. Neurosurgeons are sometimes called upon to address such unremitting pain, whether resulting from infection, stroke, amputation—or cancer. I had seen focused, destructive operations on the brain and spinal cord done for such desperate situations at the university hospital, but those sophisticated procedures had followed multiple conferences and opinions from the hospital's ethics committee.

Harold came quickly at my call. He glanced at her chart for a moment but sat with the patient and family much longer, watching and listening. His only question, asked three times in different forms, was whether her pain extended above her waist. He called his opposite number, the professor of gynecology, and again said little, asking only how soon she'd likely die. Then he returned to the bedside and offered the patient and family an operation to relieve her pain immediately by severing her cauda equina, the bundle of nerve roots that originates from the end of the spinal cord just above the belt line and controls all function in the lower body. All agreed and we went straight to the OR.

We scrubbed in silence. No black humor that day. No boxer's footwork. We began with a lumbar puncture and placed a spinal anesthetic. The dissection through shrunken muscle and diseased bone of the back was quick. We saw the blue gray membrane which enclosed the cord, the cauda equina, and the spinal fluid. Its name is dura mater, Latin for tough mother. I passed two heavy cotton ligatures around it, about one inch apart. I tied each one with extra security to avoid leakage of spinal fluid then tried to cut the dura and its contents, but my Metzenbaum scissors were too dull. Harold handed me a fresh No. 11 scalpel and I did the deed, instantly destroying every function in this woman's lower body—movement, continence, and sensation. I had never ventured so far from Hippocrates' "First, do no harm." The hour of violence we visited on this dying body left me unmoored.

I was more than reluctant to see her the next morning and left her for last on rounds. The smell in the hall was unchanged. I found her paraplegic, of course, but newly alert, comfortable and smiling, surrounded by the most grateful family I'd ever seen. I was suddenly a skilled surgeon in their eyes. I've never seen that operation described in the literature and don't expect to. She passed away in peace about one week later.

I had done my share of elective surgery by December and had by now seen many flavors of trauma. My skills were maturing. So, when the EMT crew insisted that morning that I see their patient in the ambulance before they moved him into the ER, I felt mildly curious but very confident. Until I saw him. He was a flower child about my age and gave a clear history of his illness. He'd been conversing with God in a local phone booth when God had told him to shoot himself with the speargun he'd been carrying around the city for self-defense. He'd triggered the gun with his foot, shooting himself in the head. The spear had entered his left cheek just below his eye, passing behind the eyeball and through the top of the skull, its point visible just behind his hairline and about two inches from the midline of the head, protruding about an inch from his scalp. He had no vision in his left eye but was alert and comfortable. I had been diligent in reading my journals and textbooks but had seen no literature on spear removal.

I stared from the spear to the steel floor bed of the ambulance. One of the EMTs broke the silence, suggesting that we begin by cutting off both ends of the spear to eliminate the risk of torquing it as we moved him to the OR. I mumbled agreement and we began our brain surgery in the ambulance with their bolt cutter, then moved to the OR for a relatively straightforward left frontal craniotomy to remove devitalized left frontal lobe and the midportion of the spear. Ophthalmology followed to remove the left eyeball and repair the orbit.

He was walking the halls within 48 hours, and a few days post-op had an older visitor who introduced himself as the young man's psychiatrist. He marveled that his patient's thought disorder had been so much improved by what turned out to have been a do-it-yourself frontal lobotomy. I should have named my patient as the first assistant surgeon in my dictated op note. I wondered how he had been able to afford a private psychiatrist but gradually came to understand that many of San Francisco's flower children had come from privileged families. They dressed and spoke as poor people and lived on the streets, but their orthodontia betrayed their social class to any observant ER nurse.

Having weathered the trial of SFGH, I next rotated to Moffitt to be Dr. Wilson's personal resident. I was to be the first and last face he saw each day, my only job to simplify his life. Manage his inpatients, open and close his operations, organize X-rays and lab work, dictate discharge summaries to his referring doctors. The pace of his practice verged into the realm of mania and I found myself always vigilant for disaster, never looking more than 12 hours into the future.

His mix of talent, energy, and ambition marked him as an outlier even among academic neurosurgeons. He had built a clinical and research empire and was making good on his promise to create a world-class residency training program. Malignant brain tumor—not heart attack, not pneumonia—had become the most common admitting diagnosis at this major medical center. Patients came for experimental chemotherapy from much of the western U.S. He reserved four operating rooms two days each week and did about 10 major cases on each of those days. He tried but sometimes failed to avoid elective surgery on the three "quiet" days reserved for out-patient clinic and academic pursuits. I had help now from an intern and a med student, but delegation became its own challenge and a preview of what life as a professor would be like. The volume of cases dictated that efficiency would be the coin of our realm.

He defined academic success, the pinnacle envisioned on Corey

Road. As we sat in his office at the end of one particularly trying day, he casually mentioned that he had been putting off writing a book chapter on arteriovenous malformations of the brain and now faced a publisher's deadline in two weeks. He told me to bring him a 10,000-word draft on the subject in five days to jumpstart his process. The ask was insane, but I labored through the next several nights and threw together a chaotic product, drove to his bayside home in Tiburon and handed it to him with a shudder, noting that the intricate geometry of the Persian carpet in his living room had been obscured by accumulated hair from his twin golden retrievers. I didn't fear that he'd fire me for ugly writing, but the laceration of his criticism would hurt enough.

He greeted me and looked over my draft, then, using it as an outline, became a human word processor. He spoke the finished chapter into his Dictaphone with hardly a pause, complete with footnotes and bibliography. My sentences were inverted, edited, excised. Paragraphs were moved, references quoted with stunning confidence, evidence summarized, conclusions drawn. He sounded as though he was reading something already on paper. After about 30 minutes he thanked his transcriptionist and clicked off the Dictaphone. He stood, asked about the order of his next day's cases, and saw me out as though our encounter had been entirely routine. I felt profound relief as I drove back over the Golden Gate Bridge into the city. A year later I found the textbook and confirmed that the chapter had indeed come verbatim from his Dictaphone and found that I was named as a coauthor.

His performance that night in Tiburon was unique in my experience. His fund of knowledge was profound, his surgical technique and political acumen acute. He was endlessly informed, abruptly cruel when provoked. Many of his peers avoided debating him at national meetings. But his clinical research functioned largely as a taxonomic catalog of his own cases—hundreds of pituitary tumors, malignant brain tumors, aneurysms. The ecstatic moment of discovery I'd felt looking down the barrels of my microscope at the Fernald School was compelling in a way that lists of improving surgical outcomes couldn't approach. I knew I couldn't emulate his career and that the effort would prohibit anything approaching a normal life. I did note his kids' struggles, though. He was soon to marry wife number four.

He was a short, plain man from Neosho, Missouri—his mother, like mine, ravenous for his success. His own rise had been meteoric, from Charity Hospital in New Orleans to the University of Kentucky to the chairmanship at UCSF in less than a decade. Like his peers, he'd known that neurosurgery's center of gravity, the highest rung on its academic ladder, lay at Harvard, where Harvey Cushing had invented the specialty about 70 years before. His energy was incandescent, his pedigree Appalachian. The Cushing professorship at Mass. General came open during my rotation with him and he quickly became the leading candidate. The job carried unrivaled prestige but offered less lab space, OR time, and bed capacity than he'd built in San Francisco.

It was a political snake pit, but I felt sure that he couldn't refuse the offer. I knew he was tempted. I spent many hours with him each day and couldn't miss his ambivalence. And he did take the job, but conditioned his acceptance on getting exactly those benefits of space and budget that he suspected the politics of Mass. General couldn't deliver. He didn't budge in negotiations and the MGH job went to a lesser candidate. I had just watched him step away from what he had surely coveted for much of his life. And at some level I must have taken the history lesson, begun to ask what renown might mean.

The next six months found me at the Stanford Neuropathology Lab in Palo Alto. 9 to 5. A normal life. My own bed every night. Gorgeous weather. I did undistinguished work and ate way too much pecan praline ice cream, sometimes Rocky Road for variety. Those tasty, familiar anesthetics worked well. By this point I knew a great deal about the look of various brain tumor cells and weighed 235 pounds. I was grateful to escape surgery's rigors and to enjoy this civilized schedule. To return to the OR would require finding fresh motivation, a new gear.

But I could start fresh at the beginning of my third year with my next rotation, senior resident at the university hospital. I moved from the Haight to Twin Peaks. My new apartment's panoramic Bay Bridge view offset its sketchy construction, and the walk to work through Sutro Woods was serene.

The neurosurgical service occupied the entire 8th floor, its north hall ending in a giant window looking across Golden Gate Park to the iconic bridge beyond. It was reputed among med students and staff to be a depressing unit. Many of our patients were comatose or agitated, would get well slowly if at all. Some were dangerous. One, a gigantic Samoan suffering with a malignant tumor in his hypothalamus, turned the unit into a football field whenever he escaped his restraints, aiming for immortality as he barreled toward that seductive window. Medical students didn't often seek us out and therapists of various kinds found other floors more rewarding.

My new role required some teaching, and I found myself fielding penetrating questions at the nursing station from a physical therapist named Mary. She was endlessly curious about the intricacies of the nervous system and courageous enough to work at close quarters with some of our more agitated folks. Her questions were challenging, insightful. Plus, I could answer a few. On many days I felt senior in name only, but she managed to make me feel smart. We focused narrowly on the pathologies of the nervous system. But she was very easy to look at and her voice uniquely melodic. A beauty from Big Sky Country—chocolate brown hair, deep blue eyes. She inhabited an unfailingly friendly world and was completely at ease in it. Unmistakably white.

I found myself hearing that melody of her voice in my sleep. Her smile took my breath. And miniskirts were all the rage. What began frankly as animal magnetism for me blossomed into full-blown romance. Though I'd lived in San Francisco for three years, my life hadn't included gin fizzes in Sausalito, walks to the Pacific through Golden Gate Park, or biking to Marin. My inflated body made that biking stuff a mixed blessing, but I had serious reason to persevere. I'd come three thousand miles from Corey Road, but my bunkered self had come right along, secure in the backpack of my history. Now that self could glimpse what freedom might look like, could be swept away.

I invited her as my only guest to a housewarming party on Grandview Ave. It was a first for me. I didn't think much about it at the time, but a first date masquerading as housewarming was pretty crazy. She was taken aback, I think, but too warm hearted to be suspicious. My gesture might be labeled creepy today. We talked through the night, were poles apart. My world teemed with enemies. Her reflexes were infallibly generous. Although I knew she'd grown up in Montana she seemed to hail from some distant, more empathic planet, to be the better angel of my nature. I pursued her with an urgency I hadn't known I could summon. She had just exited a difficult male entanglement and was wary of this chubby suitor. But she showed forbearance for my many shortcomings, showed a way to live better, to be better. I sorely needed her, plain as day—and I fell in love.

Dr. Wilson was a fanatical runner. His waterproof numbered bib from the Boston Marathon hung framed in his office in the company of his diplomas and academic honors. His example and my corpulence moved me to start running as a New Year's resolution on January 1, 1978. Mary said I looked green after my maiden effort, but I felt triumphant, knowing I'd covered a vast distance. I was so confident that I zeroed my odometer and drove the route, noting the comic result—0.2 miles—and rejecting it out of hand. Where was my genomic pedigree? Dad's record time at 600 yards? I would have made better time walking. But I did persist. And over the next 18 months lost 50 pounds by moving a bit more and eating a bit less.

I thrived on Mary's creative cooking. She did some running herself and introduced me to the Mediterranean Diet long before it was cool. Moussaka was a labor-intensive indulgence, but her version was far better than any other I've ever tasted, and less toxic than the Rocky Road lurking in the freezer. I wasn't yet a big person, was actually smaller, but moving up or down or sideways toward some version of adulthood. More than 40 years later I've come to understand that our bodies, these miraculous machines we all inhabit, are designed to move.

Cars are also machines, and far less miraculous. About every third autumn, Dad would briefly channel his much-younger self and spring for a new vehicle, signing for a loan at the prevailing rate of interest, and scrambling the family budget. Mom would bark, then fume. The silences across the kitchen table revealed a rare flaw in the fabric of their marital teamwork. Late in life he got his Lincoln Continental but before long was pining for a Mercedes Benz. Like most men of his time, he fully understood the hierarchy of automobiles and conveyed it faithfully to me. Many thousands of ads cemented the skill. I could name every make and model at a glance.

In 1978 I stretched my budget to breaking and bought a 1970 BMW 2500 sport sedan. My ego swelled briefly, but white smoke billowing from under the hood a few weeks later stopped me cold. Or rather, hot. I couldn't see Fell Street in front of me through the cloud of white vapor. My stomach fell through the floorboards and bounced off the asphalt. Every light on that Teutonic dashboard was alive, the engine's temperature fatally elevated. My dinner date with Mary disintegrated, followed closely by my self-esteem. I've repressed how I got the car off that busy one-way street and located Steve, a solo mechanic down the peninsula in Daly City. But I do recall clearly that my $800 monthly income was no match for a cracked cylinder head. Mary couldn't resist noting the humor of a neurosurgical resident suffering this particular injury to his car's cranium. Steve and I built an expensive ongoing relationship, and I did lots of walking over the next several weeks as I raised money for the repair and ruminated on the idea of budgeting for maintenance costs. To this day I attend closely to my car's temperature gauge.

June 1979 began my chief resident year and my job search. All of us had been well trained to be academicians and I felt confident interviewing for assistant professorships at UCLA and the University of Pittsburgh. I visited the University of Mississippi in crushing August heat. Their chairman, Robert Smith, said I could give the department major help and would have tremendous freedom to work, but that Confederate history would stifle my life in Jackson. With candor and regret he advised I look to other programs.

But the research I'd be encouraged to do in all these jobs would catalog incremental improvement in surgical outcomes and couldn't match the peak moment of discovery Reeler had yielded years before. And the ethical challenges of practice in fashionable urban markets came front of mind each Friday afternoon.

At that time, neurosurgeons in the Bay Area outnumbered those in the entire United Kingdom. Knowledge workers of every stripe craved the climate, the food, the vibe of San Francisco. These surgeons were good people, but they'd come to expect a high income and found themselves doing lots of dubious spine surgery to create it. Their numbers overwhelmed the needs of the population, and they were in the position of being able to use their advice to anxious patients to create a market for their own services, to repeal the law of supply and demand. Health care was booming and temptations to overtreat were everywhere.

Each Friday afternoon, as chief resident, I accepted patients in transfer to the university hospital who'd had surgical misadventures in the surrounding community, and who'd had no business being near the OR in the first place. The ethical pressures of an over doctored environment were plain. I had elite training and elite skills, but that pedestrian idea of supply and demand began to creep into my job search.

San Francisco offered a mirage of eternal youth. Its stunning beauty felt permanent. Seasons barely changed; children were few. I was offered a private practice job in the city, but I saw it as a postponement of adulthood, the latest extension of an already endless apprenticeship. Despite the demands of residency training, I'd dated several women during those years. But Mary was different. She was very much a grownup and now I aspired to be one too. Our romance had found its own pace, had matured over those two years. Independence, a new identity as husband, even as father, hovered in some almost graspable future. Here was an inflection point, a moment to bend the historical narrative on several axes at once. Even the ancestral imperative of relentless ascent had to be impermanent, after all. Corey Road's voice softened.

In September, my fellow resident, Isabelle, shared a recruiting letter addressed to her. It came from Topeka, Kansas. Against my ancestors' advice I arranged to meet the author, Jack Runnels, the following month at the autumn meeting of the Congress of Neurological Surgeons, a traditional venue for employers and job hunters. We said a quick hello in the meeting space but actually first spoke the next day on a hotel tennis court. We were meeting in Las Vegas, and the court threatened to melt my shoes. I'd learned the game watching Arthur Ashe and Rod Laver on TV and had worked my strokes on the east wall of the Golden Gate Park handball courts. I was a credible player, but quickly wilted in the heat. He was clearly more skillful but chose not to embarrass me.

The practice was atypical. He was employed by the Menninger Foundation, a major psychiatric hospital in Topeka. The foundation had seen a need for neurologists and neurosurgeons as far back as the 1940s, when some patients referred to them were found to have structural reasons in their brains for their psychiatric symptoms. But by 1979 those mistaken referrals were rare, and their surgeons' main focus had become the 450,000 people of Northeast Kansas.

His two senior partners had just retired almost simultaneously, and he was now on nightly ER call for all those people. He described a very busy and varied practice and extolled the logistics of small-town life. I heard about his walking to work and plentiful parking all over town. He talked about clean air and clean water and promoted the novel idea of a functioning community. I wondered whether the Menninger umbrella would offer me another layer of armor.

He was covering three ERs. The closest neurosurgeons were over an hour away in Kansas City, others more distant in Tulsa, Lincoln, and Wichita. It was obviously too much for one guy, and he told me years later that he'd have left Kansas if I hadn't joined him. He addressed my Friday afternoon ethical issue before I could raise it. "In L.A. or Pittsburgh you'd be superfluous—in Topeka you'd be necessary." That word had a reassuring ring, shorthand for big, or at least hard to despise.

I tallied the eight jobs I was considering, academic and private, into a primitive spreadsheet and spent fruitless hours trying to reason through what was an emotional problem. But Jack Runnels and Topeka were feeling right, right for the moment and right for us.

-5-
FLEDGLING PILLARS

Mary had brought home a brochure tempting us to cruise the Turkish coast and Greek islands at a bargain price. It graced our little blonde coffee table for days, an undersized placemat for our taco salad dinners, a diversion from the latest episode of MASH. One September morning I asked that the cruise become a honeymoon, a laughably timid and oblique proposal met with silence and the arched eyebrows of surprise. Our crowd of young folks had enjoyed many pleasures in San Francisco but she and I had come to know one another well over those two years. Time was passing. But marriage was a different, sobering animal—cause to be wary.

And yet, on October 27, 1979 we married at the Swedenborgian Church with 12 guests in attendance. The substitute minister's opaque German accent mangled our painstakingly-written vows. Our photographer, recruited at a bargain price from the neuropathology department, had no idea how to arrange or image living beings, leaving an irate bride to organize our guests. I felt confident in my new Ralph Lauren blue pinstripe suit until the moment of "I do," when my voice vanished and my legs quivered. I'll boast now that I could still wear that suit, long since a victim of fashion, when I donated it to a consignment shop 38 years later. I played duets at our reception with Harold, my most humane consultant. He and our guests seemed sympathetic to my many years away from the fiddle. Mary baked our cake, fresh daises atop a butter cream frosting. I remember the luscious taste as I write these words and was delighted that we could stash the leftovers into our freezer.

Mom and Dad had long been gracious to my girlfriends of whatever stripe, though they'd been especially warm to a Black dentist I'd dated a few years earlier. Several months before the wedding Mary and I invited them to Sunday morning dim sum brunch at an authentic Chinese restaurant. We were on our best behavior, anxious to make a good impression, anxious for all to go well. Each of the small, yummy dishes arrived in turn. All was fine until I signaled for the three boiled duck feet. Unadorned. Bright red.

I could have chewed that first foot all morning to no effect but could find no way to gracefully spit it out. These were molded rubber erasers disguised as food, had surely been passed over by legions of more discerning diners. Seriously underdone. Mom and Dad shared a quick glance then looked to me with unease. *Where is our accomplished son?* their eyes said. *And what has this cheerful young woman done with him?* I was speechless, gurgling to be excused and marching off to the men's room in disarray. A new generation of waiters and cooks may still hear of the crazy foreigner who finally ordered those duck feet. What my parents made of the meal I never learned.

But they could see that the missile they'd launched against the wide world in 1954 could now guide itself. I learned years later that some of Mom's family felt betrayed by our marriage. But at that moment she asked only if Mary was the love of my life. Dad busied himself with the tasks at hand and said nothing. They both in time grew to love her, found a love foreign to their hopes and bigger than their history.

We flew to Rome the next morning and literally missed the boat for our cruise in Athens after an eight-hour delay at the Rome airport, featuring many hard-eyed Italian soldiers armed with automatic weapons. The Athens harbor was deserted as night fell and the omens for us looked bleak, but Olympic Airlines found us a hotel room and flew us to Crete the next day to join the cruise.

What followed was an amazing adventure in Turkey, the Greek islands, and Rome. I skinny-dipped in the Aegean, Mary rode a camel—and suffered flea bites. Our feet spanned two continents on an Istanbul bridge. A visit to the Blue Mosque was cut short by our guide's anxiety to get Americans into his cousin's shop to buy rugs. We arrived in Rome in time for funghi season and delighted in enormous sauteed mushrooms. On Mykonos we celebrated journey's end with the crew, ate line-dried octopus, and drank too

STEEP

much Ouzo. The next morning, metabolites of alcohol combined with the diesel-choked air of downtown Athens to make a misery of our bus tour.

In November, as we newlyweds gazed from our balcony toward the Bay Bridge and the lights of the East Bay, we chewed on our future, the first big test of our union. Private practice offers in Portland, Oregon, and San Luis Obispo, California had come from unhappy surgeons and their bitter spouses. We peered through the widest lens we could muster to imagine ourselves as Kansans. To abandon San Francisco for the uncharted territory of Topeka? We were both more than skeptical. We both believed that Topeka carried real risk for a mixed-race couple. She reminded me that the KKK was reported to be active just to the east in Tonganoxie. Our friends inquired after our mental health. But we did look and were surprised to find a sophisticated medical community and an implicit invitation to grow up.

Jack had done some heavy lifting in Topeka. Much of his equipment was more modern than what I'd used in California. The ICU and nursing support were first rate. And crucially, Jack's wife Judy used her words and the story of her experience to persuade Mary that she could make a life in the Sunflower State. So, Jack and I did agree on a handshake to move in July, harboring a fantasy that Mary and I would enjoy quiet fireside chats and relish a slower pace of life in this Kansas town. We also agreed between ourselves to give the place six months. We looked at 20 houses over one manic April weekend and somehow bought a gracious colonial despite our negative net worth (something about creative financing). Meanwhile, our San Francisco landlord was offering to sell us our flimsy apartment for $20,000 more than this solid two-story Kansas house.

The departmental farewell dinner for the two graduating residents was a sumptuous affair. The humor and wine flowed freely. My departure for Oz took its share of roasting. A fellow resident gave me a bottle of the antipsychotic Thorazine as a parting gift. My reflexive smile covered the fear of stepping off the academic ladder.

But my training had been thorough, my experience broad and deep. I was ready to name myself a neurosurgeon.

The distance to Topeka would be far more than the odometer reported and the new job met with parental skepticism. But it was time to make our way in the world. We packed the car meticulously, almost as well as Dad would have done. And after a few glorious days in Mendocino County, we said goodbye to the sea and the salt air, took a last look at the Bay Bridge, and hit the road.

The BMW was as faded as its tired blue paint, and though stylish, had relied on the city's weather for its climate control. 1980 set records for heat and our puny air conditioner died halfway through Nevada. Filling the back seat were Mary's personal friends, a host of house plants. We in front acknowledged no ties to history or geography. Faulkner was wrong on that day. The past was indeed past. We aimed to be new people in this new place, a classic American strategy Dad had often pursued. We crossed the Colorado border into the endless frying pan of western Kansas, our vintage Napa wine quietly turning to toasty vinegar in the trunk. We enlisted the car's heater to cool the engine as we sprayed water onto our plants and each other. We reached Topeka's Holiday Inn at nearly midnight of our fourth day and unwound ourselves from our suddenly very foreign car. We had crossed our Rubicon and now passed through a cloud of huge flying insects circling the hotel's security lights to reach the lobby and enter our new lives. The temperature was 93 and the calendar read June 30.

We hurtled into adulthood in a single year as fledgling pillars of the community. Mary worked as a physical therapist in two local hospitals, joined the medical auxiliary, and took up horticulture. I learned that although grass is ancient, lawns are a more recent invention of the British gentry, a signal that they were as prosperous as the nobility, rich enough at least to leave some of their land uncultivated. I mowed with reluctance.

As I sat in my scrubs, inhaling an unhealthy lunch between cases that first August, a local allergist pointedly informed me that orderlies weren't allowed into the doctors' lounge and insisted that

I leave. I was startled, slow to respond—took a bite of carrot cake, glanced at my beeper, and looked up to see him being urgently chastened and pulled to a table across the room. More often I was recognized and welcomed around town as the new surgeon. My diet improved. The half gallons of pecan praline became pints and now lived for days in the freezer uneaten, but by no means forgotten.

And on April 21, 1981, our son Zack was born in the face of Mary's toxemia and our OB/GYN's hesitant relationship with her obstetrical forceps. I'd been helping Jack remove a brain tumor and had been pulled down the hall to the OB rooms. I was present but unhelpful, could catalog the major risks of this moment but struggled to grasp in my bones its gravity and wonder. I knew this baby would change my life. I could see that Zack's head had absorbed some serious hurt from those forceps, but also that his dark eyes had popped open when Mary asked that the OR lights be turned off. I cherished her survival and our new son while fretting about my new role as dad.

With our home mortgage came a need for home insurance and some inventory of our belongings. I unearthed my violin from the back of a basement closet. Our agent asked about its value. I hoped it was worth more than the one thousand dollars Mom and Dad had paid twenty years before but really had no idea. The closest dealer and appraiser, he said, was Kenneth Warren in Chicago. We took a weekend to voyage to his shop in breathless summer heat to celebrate all things Italian. Wine, food, groceries, exotic cars—and violins. His second-floor offices were hidden in a gritty neighborhood under the EL, protected by multiple locks, motion detectors, and video surveillance.

As we climbed the stairs, I was reassured by the security but uneasy that it had to be so robust. We were buzzed in and welcomed, and I opened the case on his elevated workbench. He looked closely at the fiddle from every possible angle for a full minute but chose to ignore the little rectangular paper label inside the instrument claiming the maker to be Enrico Melegari. He silently scrutinized the tail and the scroll, finally pointed out two tiny dowels I'd never noticed, inlaid into the ribs at the top and bottom of the body. "These mark the fiddle as a genuine Melegari," he said. "They probably weren't Enrico's doing. I think he got the idea from his brother, Pietro. They were self-taught, you know. The work on the scroll and the color of the varnish are consistent too. I suspect he made it late in life, based on the scroll. I'd be happy to appraise it for your insurance company."

Only then did he deign to look inside to read the maker's label and seemed almost bored by the confirmation. He looked in again, then volunteered, "Have you noticed that its sound is a bit small? The bass bar (a length of wood running the full length of the instrument inside its back) is in its original position from 1888 and that placement was chosen for playing in small spaces. I can move it if you like, and you'll notice a much fuller sound. I'll need it for a week or two and I'll FedEx it back to you in Kansas."

I was dumbfounded, instantly wary. I'd lived with this fiddle for 20 years and now this stranger knew it far better than I did, and was assuring me that he could improve it by taking it apart and subjecting it to major surgery. Not a note had been played that day, but I had to admit that its sound was small, and his expertise overwhelmed my suspicion. We agreed on the spot to leave the fiddle with him. I pointed out that the August heat was intense. Having fielded that question many times, he assured us that he wouldn't ship anything if the temperature was above 80 degrees. Before we left, he toured us through his shop, packed with stringed instruments in various states of convalescence. He drew our particular attention to "Mr. Ma's cello." We passed through the motion detectors and re-entered the heat of the afternoon.

As we walked toward our hotel I wondered about self-taught Enrico and his brother, remembered the flinty thrift of Corey Road, began to grasp that this instrument meant more than I'd guessed. Of course it had fueled a social climb. But it also was an amulet of parental love, might even open a path toward some kind of peace. Still, it rarely left its case for the next 20 years.

Our new home, this capital city of 130,000, lacked art house theaters. Asian and European cuisines had not reached our corner of the Great Plains. Alcohol was unavailable for public sale on Sundays. But life's logistics began to roll easy for the new parents. Every destination was close. Lots more space than people, more asphalt than cars. Understandably, Jack had disappeared for two weeks as soon as I'd learned where the ORs and bathrooms were. I was suddenly Eastern Kansas' senior neurosurgeon, the stakes high, my decisions final. I was also Eastern Kansas' only neurosurgeon, a lonely posting. There were moments when I sorely missed my professors' oversight and was reminded more than once that academic credentials don't create good judgment or control what's professionally euphemized as brisk bleeding.

One of my first office patients that summer brought her anxiety with her into the exam room. A middle-aged brown-skinned woman dressed for an important event, sporting a church-ready hat—definitely unhappy changing into a hospital gown. Her eyes were more than cautious, veered toward suspicion. I moved slowly, spoke short English words. I wrote her history as she related it. She had had surgery five years before for a ruptured lumbar disc. Now the leg pain was back, far worse than before. Her study suggested a large new rupture. We agreed to go to the OR.

The dissection was treacherous. No familiar landmarks. No reassuring professors. Her scar was thick and dense, but below it somewhere lay her flattened nerve root. I navigated with patience and with full attention, my CV shelved. I removed the disc fragment and relieved her unhappy nerve root. She was delighted. And because she was a busy beautician, her delight reached many ears.

My surgical skills developed far more quickly than would have occurred in any academic setting, thanks to the volume and variety of the cases I faced. Word of mouth overwhelmed what any marketing firm could have imagined. I grew in expertise. But each day I gave thanks for my professors and fellow residents who had modeled how to operate, but also how to behave. How to move, to speak, to not speak, to touch. How to dampen fear. I'd been an apprentice for six years, absorbing all this by osmosis.

Case volume brought skill and weariness in equal measure. Jack and I weren't roused from sleep for trivia, but even the most experienced and tactful night nurses couldn't fully silence that phone 18 inches from my ear, its summons recurring every other night. So, in 1982 we recruited Khadyampatti Arjunan as our third surgeon and instantly improved the quality of our lives by a third. 15 nights each month wedded to the phone shrank to 10. Aptly named for Krishna's charioteer in the *Bhagavad Gita*, he was indeed a prince, and a compassionate physician.

1982 also brought my oral board exam, what was to be my last formal academic test: three hours of questioning divided equally among neurology, spinal surgery, and cranial surgery. Success would mean "board certification," full membership in the neurosurgical guild. I studied, submitted my case experience, and traveled to Rochester, Minnesota for the ordeal. I sailed through the first two and a half hours, then stumbled in managing a case of pediatric head trauma presented to me by the professor and chairman of neurosurgery at the University of Alabama. And failed the exam.

My crowning gold star had been withheld. As I look back, it's clear that the injury he described was inevitably fatal, either from hemorrhage or from brain swelling, depending on the surgeon's decisions. But during his questioning my anxiety had edged toward panic as I tried to rescue an increasingly desperate situation. Not a good look for the examiners.

Anger had filled every crevice of Corey Road, had been my lifelong companion. Original equipment. I've just recently made friends with it and have learned that it instantly and reliably overtakes me in the wake of potent fear, a fear that I don't count, don't even exist. The fear always comes first, the anger then follows slowly—or quickly. So now the examiner had enraged my younger self. He had been the quintessential Southern gentleman, and I leaped to judge him as too much a white man of his place and time, to judge him as he likely had judged me. I might have been right, but I was also utterly disabled in the cab to the airport, unable to loosen my jaw or unglue my shoulders from my earlobes.

STEEP

But by some alchemy I turned rage to resolve during that flight home. Baldwin's right about history's control being unconscious—I dredged a sliver of my past into full view that night. I channeled my ancestors, resurrected Mr. McCormick from that afternoon at the Latin School years before. During our descent into Kansas City, I put up my tray table and that day's fear with it.

I set up a nook in our basement and despite demands of practice, fatherhood, and marriage, gave at least two hours each evening for the next 360 days to the goal of knowing more than any examiner about any point he might choose to raise. The result spoke for itself. The following year in New Orleans I came second in a group of 75 applicants. My final gold star arrived, the present moment finally a place to bask. But I had so long distrusted the here and now that I couldn't enjoy it without help. I celebrated with far too much fine wine at a storied restaurant in the French Quarter and was fortunate to reach my hotel room unmugged, my wallet secure in my pocket.

November 2, 1983, brought our second son, Christopher. Mary's toxemia came sooner now and was more severe, manifested by dangerously-abnormal kidney and liver functions, more than justifying the little foil-wrapped IV bottle of nitroprusside that dampened her insanely high blood pressure from one instant to the next. Her pregnancy had climaxed as a threat to her life. This couldn't be Mary in that bed.

I knew much too much. As I scanned the monitors and looked at the labs, I could credibly imagine her death. The dread receded with effort and with love, that little meaningful word. Chris arrived three weeks early with respiratory distress and came home, too soon, on his third day of life—his doctors overly-reliant on our medical knowledge. We did give his breathing close attention and tag-teamed the suctioning duties. Mother and son survived. But it might well have been otherwise.

We gradually settled into a privileged life. I practiced medicine while Mary multitasked: volunteering, managing our home, teaching neurology to physical therapy assistant students at a local college. She was a gifted PT and reluctant to leave the profession, her choice stealing part of who she was. Mostly we set about being our new selves, now parents and homeowners, reweaving our corner of the town's fabric day by day. We aimed to build a life that spoke for us; however the winds of national history and politics blew.

But our Bay Area self-image died hard in those early years. Away from Topeka we were quick to mention San Francisco and slow to be Kansans. In 1988, eager to teach residents, I interviewed for assistant professor jobs in Ann Arbor and Portland, Oregon, quickly learning that my lack of recent publications would relegate me to entry-level roles and the backwaters of academic politics. The die really had been cast in 1980. So, I learned to enjoy teaching whoever wanted to learn, especially patients and families. Meanwhile, I had more work than I could do, and that work came front of mind each morning. Results and ethics were strong, real vindication for our move to Oz. I hadn't needed the Thorazine, reaching instead for a sense of place.

But we were offered a glamorous lifeline in the autumn of 1984, a respite from our little town. The chairman of neurosurgery at Howard University told me he was creating a neurosurgical service on the island of St Thomas, to be staffed by Black surgeons from the mainland, and invited me to join the rotation. We could choose our two-week period of service. My time would be donated but his grant would cover our housing. This decision was not hard. We'd escape the Kansas winter for an exotic family vacation, and I'd frolic in the ocean! At last, my skills would be recognized, no, celebrated.

We chose the last two weeks of February and prepared for major travel with two busy little boys. We landed at Charlotte Amalie, the capital, and looked for our designated driver. The wait was long, but the boys entertained themselves romping and rolling on the airport's dirt floor, rich with local micro-organisms.

After more than a few calls our driver appeared, a thin young man busy with many hustles. He welcomed us with a brassy voice and opened the back door of his van with some ceremony, while evaluating our clothing and humdrum luggage. He quickly got us to our housing, a classic tropical bungalow smelling of suntan lotion,

STEEP

insecticide, and mildew, but mostly of bleach. I'm sure our tip was judged inadequate. I made my way to the hospital early the next morning and was relieved to hear from Margaret, the head nurse, that I wouldn't be going to the OR although they had a reasonable supply of surgical instruments. Not enough nurses. She was stout and loud, long suffering, and very much in charge—steeped in local knowledge, a skillful navigator of island bureaucracy. She toured me through the hospital and proudly showed me its latest piece of equipment, a Siemens polytomogragh, ideal for improving on the accuracy of ordinary X-rays, especially useful for subtle neck fractures. It was far more advanced than what we had in Topeka, and I couldn't help wondering who had paid for it.

I was to carry a beeper, see emergencies, and staff an outpatient clinic. The beeper resembled a gray paperweight invested with a fine layer of dust. It looked and felt like a brick. I resolved to keep it close at all times. As we tested it, its speaker produced a mournful cackle of static followed by a tangled version of Margaret's voice. I feared that I would miss a flow of critical calls, but this weighty tool remained resolutely silent day after day.

We enjoyed the beach each morning, but our boys redefined my experience. Chris was a fearless 15-month-old explorer, insisting wordlessly and persistently that he could walk unharmed into the sea and make his way to Europe on foot. He delighted in being pulled from Caribbean waves flowing over his head. We grabbed whatever body part we could feel, typically a well-toned arm. When he tired of strolling the ocean floor he'd practice grabbing and throwing handfuls of fine white sand. This exercise of grasp and release charmed us, but our neighbors, a group of well-oiled, tanning New Yorkers, found no amusement in his joyful sandstorms.

After several days of radio silence, I began to wonder about my beeper's viability and about my role, especially as we read in each morning's paper about the major traumas of the previous night. Car wrecks were a big hazard for partying tourists here, but I wasn't in the loop. Margaret patiently assured me that all major emergencies (especially for tourists) were airlifted to Miami or San Juan.

At my first outpatient clinic I reviewed each patient's chart before I saw them, discouraged that these records needed both hands to lift, their organization unfathomable to my eye. But my patients saved the day. Each had memorized their entire history—medicines, allergies, illnesses, operations. Everything. They were walking medical records, an oral culture of health care. Each in turn leaned forward to whisper that they didn't trust the local doctors and that in any serious situation their last word would be Miami. They had adapted skillfully to island reality but were grateful for my attention. I had little to offer them. My skills were fine, just irrelevant.

I carried my beeper everywhere, careful to keep it dry even as I showered, wedging it behind the head. We'd heard that the neighboring island of St. John was exquisite, but the 30-minute boat ride seemed irresponsibly long. After 13 silent days I finally surrendered to the lure of its tropical beauty, and we set off. The beeper crackled to life just as we disembarked; "emergency" its only recognizable word. I turned and left Mary and the boys, got back on the boat for the return trip.

I reached the ER to find a real case on this, my last working day. A seven-year-old girl had fallen and complained of neck pain, her head torqued about 30 degrees to the left. Plain X-rays suggested but didn't clearly show a fracture of the second cervical vertebra. She was okay neurologically and was protected by a hard collar. Just the moment for their brand-new polytomograph! I started to wheel my patient to X-ray, but Margaret promptly curbed my enthusiasm. Only "George" knew how to operate the machine, and he worked on Thursdays, making his real money during the rest of the week chartering deep sea fishing trips. Today was Friday. I shuffled back to the ER in frustration and embarrassment to break the news to the girl's mom. She was well ahead of me, though. She was sympathetic but had already booked their flight to Miami.

Because I had more time on my hands than I'd expected, I was tempted each afternoon by the tourist retail scene. Little Switzerland offered beautiful watches at duty-free prices, and I fell for a battery-driven Rolex, with its unique steel and gold band. The company was fearful of Japanese competition in those years and had introduced this entry level model in something of a panic. It didn't sell well, and Rolex soon stopped its production, but quickly righted itself with its traditional self-winding models.

It would be my latest layer of armor, literally a wristband announcing membership in some rarefied club. It looked gorgeous on St Thomas, less so in Topeka. I couldn't tell whether anyone admired it, resented it, or even noticed it, but before long I recognized it as textbook conspicuous consumption—a cultural obstacle, far out of place in my plainspoken workspace. It boasted many features but lacked an off switch for my ancestral treadmill. Today it sits in its saddle brown leather box waiting patiently to validate its owner.

I was known to change a diaper and take out the trash, was capable of refilling the dish detergent dispenser. I made friends with our Kirby vacuum cleaner though I needed both hands to budge it. But our home's division of labor has eroded my memory of our sons' early years. Mary wakened for crying boys. I roused for ER calls. I remember holidays and family vacations, and did get to most parent-teacher conferences, school plays, and soccer games, but too often only my body showed up. Attention is a finite resource and neurosurgery was always hungry for mine.

Our path had taken us far from the coasts and the academy, but my parents followed. They had long wanted to live in San Francisco and moved there during my residency. They came next to Broken Arrow, Oklahoma in 1983 to be closer to their grandsons. Each move came with a new federal engineering job for Dad but also kept us close. After his retirement in 1985 they moved to Topeka. We were knit tight.

I was their wellspring of pride and identity, but their hopes and fears lived on. Mom once confided that to get competent medical care she'd need to leave Topeka for a real academic medical center. She reminded me that they'd always hoped for a son who flew to international consultations in his Learjet, in the next breath admonished me to work less hard. They were firmly enclosed by their own past and imagined that my climb would have some blissful summit, that infinite success could come—and be maintained—without effort. They were hardly alone in their magical thoughts. I showed filial piety and held my tongue. Our affection had long been hooked to desire. Mine to satisfy, theirs to be vindicated.

They seemed immortal until the spring of 1987 when I saw Mom's massively enlarged heart on a chest X-ray from Oral Roberts University Hospital. The diagnosis was viral cardiomyopathy. Her energy declined with her cardiac output, but I was too blinkered to see the pace of her illness. She was a fan of Ralph Waldo Emerson's essay "Self-Reliance," skeptical of sweeping social ideologies and political movements, but determined to help build America's more perfect union. She imagined funding a college scholarship for Black graduates from Topeka High and the idea found its way into her will. Mary later convinced Dad to fund it while he was alive so that he could meet the first few winners. Each of those meetings brought a sparkle to his eyes.

Dad found her on their bedroom floor on April 7 but couldn't imagine her dead and called Mary for advice. The EMTs hustled her reflexively to one of those ER cubicles I'd so often occupied. I sprinted from the OR to find her body enduring futile chest compressions, her belly inflated from a misguided attempt at intubation. My shock stopped time and erased memory. Past and future disappeared. I had learned too well to deny hurt in the service of performance. Now that restraint could not hold me together. My layers of armor vaporized in the heat of that instant. This pain had no name. Like a leafless tree in midwinter, alive but undressed, I was fixed in place, catatonic in body and mind, without memory for the following days—the gathering of distant family, the memorials, the condolences.

We were overrun with covered dishes and compassion from much of the town. Every horizontal surface in our home overflowed with flowers and letters, some from folks I barely knew. The community Jack had described years before revealed its reality in this hard moment. I was singed by a biblical love, a love like a refiner's fire. I was unable to speak at her memorial and ineffective for weeks, stumbling back toward something like normalcy over the next many months. But Dad had it worse. As ever, he was compelled to act and to move—to donate her clothing, to sell their house, and to remarry too soon.

The blank time brought no flash of insight, only a pull to persist with life. Chris and Zack drew my attention. They didn't stop growing up, and our neighborhood suited them well. Many playmates, a short walk to a good public school. We played driveway tennis; they endured the usual driveway bike traumas. Chris skipped training wheels and Zack chose First Congregational Church for our family.

In 1991 an upstairs leak collapsed our kitchen ceiling. As we reoccupied the room, we noted that our boys were growing but our space was not. The wallpaper of this suddenly much too cozy room took more than its share of dings. We needed a larger kitchen, but after seeing the remodeling estimates actually wound up in a larger house two blocks away. Ironically, our new home featured a truly tiny butler's kitchen in need of demolition. This gracious colonial, built in 1933, hovered at some threshold of ostentation, was the house my parents had always craved. Its original deed featured a restrictive covenant, forbidding the owner from selling to Negroes or Jews. Effective in its day, though unenforceable since 1948. Its original specifications boasted of lead pipes and asbestos insulation.

Mary and I drove off to our separate errands that crisp December morning years later, holidays on our horizon. An hour later she returned to find a phalanx of three squad cars at our curb, another blocking the driveway, a growing collection of curious neighbors buzzing on the front lawn. I came a few minutes later, walked a few steps up the driveway, more ready for fight than flight. I was blocked by a cop as tall as our front door and nearly as wide and refused entry into our own house. He barked about "clearing the scene" and had no interest in my ID. This would be a losing battle in every way.

After a very long 15 minutes, a sergeant stepped briskly out our front door to explain that we'd had a break-in and that his team had been searching room to room for intruders. My gut relaxed a fraction. Someone (or more than one someone) had come through our back yard and torqued our French doors from their hinges, smashing the glass to reach our living room—and had been instantly repelled by the primal scream of our security alarm. They'd been within sight of my fiddle parked in its open case, easily our most valuable possession. Most of the broken glass littered the floor, but I delicately swept a few tiny shards from the red varnish of my old companion. We found nothing missing after a search from basement to attic. The fiddle was likely unfenceable, its varnish mercifully unmarked. I went for the dustpan and broom.

The sergeant explained their break-in protocol. No homeowners present simplified his search and protected everybody. He assured us our house was unoccupied, wrote a complex case number onto a form, and presented it to me with a touch of ceremony. So, I was in that moment a truly big person, had climbed far enough from Corey Road to be robbed. "These things peak just before Christmas," he confided. "It's all the ads for stuff people don't have money to buy." His wife, it turned out, had been a patient, and had done well.

Radio chatter called them to move on. Our neighbors dispersed to their Saturday mornings. I looked at the multiple letters and digits of our case number and asked the sergeant whether he could envision a lower priority for his force's ongoing attention. His tiny smile was eloquent. I wondered how we'd fix the French doors.

Our gracious home required many renovations over many months. As plaster dust fell onto our makeshift basement dining table we fled to a local motel. Mary designed our new kitchen while wrangling busy kids and dismissive contractors. Once, home late, I approved a design change that she had rejected earlier in the day. Our contractor had tempted "doc" to leave his lane, a mistake I did not repeat. We learned from Don Hall, whose dad had built the house, that below its foundation lay a number of tractor parts and other abandoned farm tools. Years later, Chris somehow found a 250-millimeter World War I artillery shell embedded behind our basement drywall. He wedged it into his backpack and presented it to his third grade class for show and tell. He wasn't jailed and the story didn't make national news, but we all agreed that bombs (even disarmed ones) shouldn't go to school.

My psyche remained firmly in Filene's basement as we crept toward affluence. In some years we almost obeyed my parents' rule of thirds, living on a third of our income, saving a third, and paying the rest in taxes. I knew nothing about investing but was resolved not to be stupid with what now felt like real money, though the garrulous financial wizards in the doctors' lounge were difficult to ignore. Competence remained vital to self-image. After way too much thought we bought a few stocks but had just enough sense to find financial planners too. They insisted on something called asset allocation and promptly sold most of what we'd bought. A downturn in 1987 quieted the lounge wizards and confirmed our planners' judgment. But before all their strategic advice came Mom's rule of thirds.

The practice hummed but our employer, the Menninger Foundation, was coming under increasing pressure from managed care. Open-ended payment for inpatient psychiatry was coming to an end. Meanwhile, Jack was struggling with depression in the wake of a horrific malpractice lawsuit and had moved to Palo Alto to banish his demons, taking an academic position at Stanford's Santa Clara VA Hospital. Senior Menninger administrators chose this moment to call Arjunan and me to a meeting, where their byzantine accounting made it obvious to them that we were greatly overpaid and would need to take a major pay cut to remain within the Menninger family.

We met at a long table, three smiling white money men in sober, well-fitted suits facing two dark-skinned guys in olive-green surgical work clothes. They patronized us with unusual finesse but struggled to conceal their hunger for cash flow. Still, we hesitated. We knew nothing about running a small business and life under the foundation's umbrella had been comfortable. But our time had come. With real anxiety we elected to leave the "family" in 1990 and launch a private practice. The Menninger Foundation chose not to adapt to its new reality and ultimately left for Houston. Our new practice's accounting was clear, though rudimentary. I shed a layer of institutional armor, felt lighter. Overhead plunged.

-6-
PEAKS & VALLEYS

One Wednesday afternoon in 1986 found me in our driveway surrounded by the usual collection of bikes, trikes, and Cozy Coupes. The traffic cop was Ryan, a boisterous red-haired five-year-old who lived next door. The dozen or so undersized motorists headed home for dinner, and I looked forward to a quiet evening before the next day's surgery schedule. As I was brushing my teeth, Ryan's Mom called to say that he had just cried out and grabbed his head, and now wouldn't move his left arm. By the time I got dressed and next door he was hard to keep awake.

We all piled into our cars and hustled to the ER. CT showed a plum-sized blood clot in his right temporal lobe, with an irregularity at its inner margin. We didn't have time for special studies to demonstrate it, but those black squiggles looked like a collection of abnormal blood vessels, an arteriovenous malformation. These malformations don't nourish the surrounding brain—they consist of a nest of small arteries connected directly with local veins. No intervening capillary bed to slow blood flow or reduce pressure in those thin-walled draining veins. The bleeding had likely arisen from the rupture of one of these veins and the clot had now shifted the brain from right to left, creating his neurologic deficit and demanding immediate attention. My partner, Arj, was on call and we both took Ryan to the OR.

I was well aware as we scrubbed that our patient lived next door, but Ryan lost something of his identity once the surgical drapes, monitors, and catheters were in place. There is ceremony in draping a surgical field, a ritual that quiets the mind. The drapes revealed an expanse of scalp and erased my neighbor. Our attention turned from Ryan to his problem and stayed put there for the next three hours. We made our standard question mark incision into his right temporal scalp and began our night of work.

Because the clot was large and came almost to the cortical surface it wasn't hard to find, and we quickly began removing it. The challenge would come at its bottom, where we'd need to be alert for the malformation. Without an arteriogram (that special X-ray study) we'd need to move with particular care to find and cut its feeding arteries first. If we cut the draining veins first, local arterial pressure would rise, making for serious blood loss and a much longer night. So, as we approached the clot's inner boundary, we slowed our pace and brought in the operating microscope, knowing that with the clot mostly removed, the pressure in Ryan's head had fallen to normal and we had no further need for haste.

Our micro instruments tiptoed along the inner boundary of that clot for what seemed like half an hour until a smallish artery slipped into view. It coursed laterally, straight at us, nestled in a bundle of engorged, red veins. We burned it with our bipolar coagulator to interrupt blood flow through it, then burned it again for insurance, turning it nearly to charcoal. We dealt with two more arteries in the same way. As we closed those arteries the swollen veins slowly shrank, turned from scarlet to magenta to indigo, then reassuringly to black from lack of flow. We cut the arteries, then the veins, and rolled the spherical malformation gently into the cavity where the clot had been, then into our specimen dish for Pathology.

We finished in the early hours of the morning and my black Saab had the road to itself for the five-minute drive home. As I stood in our driveway, now empty of kids and vehicles, I looked up into a brilliant, moonless night sky and smelled woodsmoke nearby. A Santa Fe train whistle broke the stillness with its usual G major 6th chord, its cars passing across the Great Plains to some unknown destination. I was a world away from the brilliant lights, the blood and cacophony of an hour before, and took a moment to inhale Topeka's unassuming beauty. I looked up at the infinity of stars and thought about this climb toward ever-greater renown, wondered whether the ascent would ever end, whether I'd ever be big enough. But for that moment I'd achieved my proper size and fit neatly through our back door. I'd done a good turn for my neighbor—and had been reminded that life and death lived right next door.

I made my standard goodnight call to the recovery room from our kitchen. Ryan was waking up well, moving all four limbs to command. Labs looked good. It was a little after 3. The sun would soon rise on a new day of surgery.

As usual, I'd brought my vigilance home and was slow to re-enter its familiar spaces. Lying down would be easy, sleep less so. I'd be up before 6, but wouldn't use an alarm clock, hadn't needed one since I'd worn that wristwatch to the playground decades before. The passage of time had made its way into my cells. Ryan recovered beautifully and, though the clot deprived him of some peripheral vision to his left, he was able to adapt with a reflexive head turn and ultimately become an architectural engineer. A big win for the home team.

I hadn't yet joined those fuzzy big people I'd imprinted from our first TV set but did bring my best game to a much smaller audience in 1993. We had admitted a middle-aged man with a hemorrhage from an aneurysm of the anterior communicating artery. He was alert but his neck was rigid because the fresh blood had inflamed the membranes and spaces around his brainstem and upper spinal cord. His headache was terrific. Our practice saw about 15 to 20 ruptured aneurysms each year and this location wasn't unusual.

What was unusual was that he had had surgery for that same aneurysm (about the size of a swollen pea) two weeks before in a neighboring state. His hair had barely begun to grow back. Our arteriogram showed that the previous surgeon's clip, intended to lie across the aneurysm's neck and isolate it from the circulation, was instead perched askew high on its dome, leaving the neck (or base) unclipped and the source of this new bleed. These titanium clips resemble spring loaded bobby pins—just much smaller and stronger. They come in many shapes and sizes, ranging from just 5 millimeters (0.2 inches) up to an inch long, machined for precision and for decades of closing strength far greater than arterial blood pressure.

My first unspoken impulse was to steer clear of this deadly

situation, to insist that the first surgeon deal with his own complication. But moving him made no sense and this man wanted to stay in Topeka, to risk his life with this total stranger. He wouldn't be the first or last of my patients to show such bravery. We cleared the schedule. My partner John Ebeling would help me take this on.

Arterial bleeding within the skull lasting more than a few seconds takes up lots of space very quickly and kills about 15 percent of these patients before they can reach a hospital. But most bleeds are very brief. Blood rushes to fill spaces between the brain and skull and between the lobes of the brain. Many bleeds are caused by rupture of an aneurysm, a local area of thinning and bulging of an artery's wall. Most aneurysms arise from five connected arteries at the center of the base of the brain, the so-called circle of Willis, a bit smaller in diameter than a silver dollar and shaped more like a tiny pentagon. One of the five, the anterior communicating artery, connects the main arteries supplying the right brain with those supplying the left, allowing blood to cross from one hemisphere to the other and offering a chance for recovery to many stroke victims who suffer a blockage of a right or left-sided artery.

This anterior communicator, no more than 15 millimeters long, lives in the midline of the head, about three inches straight back from the bridge of the nose. To reach it requires painstaking dissection of the frontal lobe away from the temporal lobe, creating a path down to the artery and the aneurysm. This second bleed would aggravate the brain's fragility, would require taking extra pains.

I was discouraged but not surprised to see that the first surgeon had approached from the right, a path mechanically easier for right-handed surgeons. I would have done the same. Approaching from the left was slightly more awkward and endangered vital functions of the dominant hemisphere—the ability to speak, write, and understand language. Either approach would go through fresh blood and older, more tenacious clot. But coming from the left would at least take us through unoperated anatomy and might allow us to see the unclipped bottom of the aneurysm and the left side of its neck before we had to see and maybe manipulate the previous clip. So, we'd approach from the left, the C-shaped scalp incision beginning just in front of the ear and ending above the left eye and just behind the hairline.

The final bit of microdissection around an aneurysm is much like bomb disposal, but today just reaching the bomb would require a finesse that defines our specialty's public brand, would require hours of grace under mounting duress. We picked our way through surprisingly dense scar and blood, separating the frontal and temporal lobes millimeter by millimeter. We sighted the left internal carotid artery as it emerged from the base of the skull. Its flow enables language. Serious care required. Just ahead was the anterior cerebral artery, which would lead us to our bomb.

If our progress to this point had been slow, we now downshifted to glacial. The operating microscope, invented in Vermont in 1967, was our indispensable ally. It stood patiently like a silent seven-foot-tall stork wrapped in transparent, sterile plastic, then rolled up to the OR table like the perfectly-balanced 500-pound helper it was. It gave us stunning clarity and magnification, light more brilliant than the light of day. With a tiny adjustment of the self-retaining retractor (a bit like a skinny lockable slinky) on the frontal lobe, we caught a glimpse of titanium—the tips of the previous clip. To this point we hadn't been exactly casual but circulating nurses from other rooms had been slipping in and out to lend or borrow equipment while Beethoven played from the boombox.

Now we sealed the room. Our circulating nurse taped signs to the glass of the OR doors reading "Do Not Enter" in large block letters. The music stopped. We had two pints of blood in the room, four more in the blood bank.

We stepped back to look once more at the arteriogram, to judge where exactly the unclipped portion of the aneurysm lay relative to the clip. Then we inched ahead to find the origin of the anterior communicator and tiptoed medially to see—finally—our adversary. Swirling arterial blood was clearly visible through its gossamer walls. I read those eddies as sinister, a menace to our effort. I had done calamitous aneurysm surgery and knew all too well this particular face of sudden death. The previous clip was untouchable, but very much in our way. I was able to operate for only a minute or two at a time, then stop to breathe. I wonder how many surgeons hold their breath at such moments, a habit that erodes coordination and performance.

Emotional restraint was crucial now, a kind of dissociation mined from Corey Road. We found a tiny space in front of the aneurysm, then struggled through scar tissue on its back side. We looked for threadlike perforating arteries coursing away from us back from the communicator. We did see a few, but had we seen them all? Injuring those could leave our patient unable to speak or move.

Our micro dissectors picked persistently at the scar. At last, a sliver of empty space opened behind the aneurysm. I exhaled, turned to collect myself and to look at the choice of clips. Many possibilities —long, short, curved, straight. I chose one barely longer than a grain of rice. I wasn't able to call for the clip applier at the moment of truth —the stress had robbed me of speech. It appeared in my hand in its proper position of function thanks to Lil Thompson, our serene and experienced scrub nurse. My left hand advanced that 7-millimeter straight clip across the neck. Time vanished. I released the clip's jaws — and abruptly the aneurysm was no more, now a deflated and inert bit of fibrous tissue. Ebeling declared he'd never seen anything like it and broke into gloved applause. I too had never seen anything like it. Our anesthesiologist was understandably relieved. The circulating nurse turned on some triumphal music for closing. The aneurysm's collapse gave us space to see the right-sided vessels across the midline. We removed the previous clip.

It was a major triumph before a tiny, knowledgeable audience, but more a mission accomplished in that moment than a life saved. We had erased the immediate danger to this man's life but had no assurance that he would wake. His risk of major stroke in the next week was one in four, his risk of death still one in twenty.

The coming evening's work took no note of our peak moment. The signs on the OR windows came down, replaced by a blizzard of yellow Post-it notes telling me about consults to see and lab work to check before I left for home.

I was slow to re-enter my reality, suspended in some state of grace. The alarms and monitors of the recovery room barked and bayed more than usual, vying in discordance and volume for the nurses' attention. As I wrote post-op orders, I took close note of my penmanship and of the nurse's scarlet fingernail polish as she connected my patient's lines and monitors. My locker's combination took a long moment to recall, and my belt buckle seemed to belong to someone else.

Our patient made a perfect recovery, and I did complete that evening's work. As I turned the door handle and walked in on the day's last hospital consult, I met the wide eyes of my latest fearful patient surrounded by his posse of uneasy family, all more than ready to see the doctor after far too long a wait.

The audience had indeed been small. No press conference, no entourage. My mind's eye roamed back into that operating room, peering under the drapes and behind the anesthesia machine, looking for those elusive big people. I'd just now come from Hamilton's "room where it happened." I was Teddy Roosevelt's "man in the arena," wet with sweat, eyeglasses smudged with dust and blood from my patient's skull. This drama had had a solitary author, had been a first and only draft. No chance to revise the text or spin the ending. But now my mind found itself in an empty, sterile space. The room had shrunk, was silent, not yet re-sterilized. I too was smaller than an hour before. And the whispers of "not good enough" would not cease.

Operating rooms are arenas filled with existential drama, but they're also workplaces filled with rivalries and alliances, romance and gossip. The rhythm of any given case ebbs and flows. Circulating nurses chat about their kids. I was known to tell a joke or two. Anesthesia glances away from the automatic alarms of their monitors to scan *The Wall Street Journal*, earning a reprimand from the scrub nurse. There are debates about whether to play music, about what can be agreed upon. There were days when I preferred the company to the work.

I'd had a far different experience with aneurysm surgery years earlier. On a Saturday morning in 1983, a local law school student was brought to the ER after collapsing with a sudden headache. He roused only to shouted voice, but once awake, could manage a normal neurologic exam—oriented, moving his limbs to command. His CT scan showed a major hemorrhage, and arteriogram revealed an aneurysm an inch in diameter at the tip of the basilar artery. Its back side smooth, its front knobbled and irregular.

This was by definition a giant aneurysm, and it was living in the most dangerous spot in the head. I asked my partner Jack to help me decide what to do. Surgical mortality for aneurysms in this location had been 100% until the 1970s. Without surgery patients always rebled, their life expectancy about six months. They'd been considered inoperable until a gifted and courageous Canadian, Charles Drake, devoted his career to the problem, analyzing in painstaking and painful detail the failures of each of his first 12 surgical cases as he began to establish the conditions necessary for success.

With experience and time, 100% became 25%. Statistics began to accumulate and to guide surgical decision making. An alert patient with a small hemorrhage (and a small aneurysm) was more likely to survive. Early surgery avoided the risk of rebleeding within the first week and reduced the risk of stroke. Adequate exposure— room to operate so deep in the brain—had been a major problem. He had addressed it with several techniques, including drainage of spinal fluid from the lumbar spine during surgery, diuretics, hyperventilation by anesthesia, drainage of spinal fluid from the ventricular system of the brain itself. All aimed to shrink the brain, allowing more gentle retraction and giving the surgeon more room to see and work at the center of the head. Even under ideal conditions, a surgical mortality of one-in-four was sobering, but preferable to death in six months.

STEEP

Our patient's sleepy state, the size of the aneurysm, and the large volume of hemorrhage argued against him, but youth was in his favor. Jack had done a number of basilars, and as a resident I'd made several dissections down to the location for Dr Wilson. We spoke frankly with the family. They asked that we go ahead, and we began in the early afternoon.

The opening was routine. We were prepared for rupture of the aneurysm. Two pints of blood in the room, four more in the blood bank. We shrank the brain with every technique known, but the right temporal lobe remained seriously swollen and lifting it enough to glimpse the aneurysm's territory was a struggle. With time and patience, though, we inched through the fresh clot to see the basilar artery. With a bit more retraction we glimpsed the base of the aneurysm. We couldn't expect to see all of it given its size but felt we could get a clip across its neck through the exposure we had. Picture working through a small funnel, its tip cut off, creating space enough to admit a walnut. A few more minutes of very tense dissection showed us the back of the neck. I could pass a straight micro dissector fully behind it, past midline.

But my first move to define the front of the neck ruptured the aneurysm and created our worst nightmare. I'd never seen so much blood come so fast from such a tiny surgical field. It was moving fast enough for us to hear it hiss through our suckers. The field vanished. No anatomy was visible, only a torrent of arterial blood.

But we weren't defeated. We changed from micro suckers to much larger ones to clear the field. The anesthesiologist gently reduced the blood pressure, began transfusing, and called for more blood to be sent and crossmatched. But a lack of working space gradually became a major problem. We had just enough room to work under bloodless circumstances, but now not quite enough. I had placed a piece of anticoagulant foam and a tiny cotton sponge to seal the site of the rupture, but with two large suckers and all the anticoagulant materials in place we just had too little room to work.

Also, our mechanical efforts to stop the bleeding were failing. It felt as though the entire front face of the aneurysm had torn away, upward and out of reach. We'd apply gentle local pressure at the rupture site for several minutes at a time, but each time we irrigated with saline and ever so carefully eased the cotton sponges away, the torrent resumed. Two pints, four pints, six pints. We had now replaced the patient's blood volume completely and were still not seeing the front of the aneurysm's neck.

Jack suggested that we put a temporary clip on the trunk of the basilar artery itself so that we could get a better shot at seeing the front of the neck in a less-bloody field. I agreed. We had little choice, although we both knew that placing that clip on the basilar could well produce a fatal brain stem injury. We hoped to quickly place a second permanent clip more superiorly to collapse the aneurysm specifically, then remove the temporary clip. But more superior clips made no impact on the bleeding. We were finally forced to accept a clip placement on the basilar that would certainly kill this kid. We had controlled his bleeding at the cost of his life.

The room felt especially frigid now. I'd been in a cold sweat for an hour and now shivered intermittently as we closed. We didn't speak. The boombox was silent. Our patient did not waken and declined to brain death in 24 hours. His family struggled with this catastrophe but were gracious amid their tears. Sudden death is always a shock, especially when it comes to the young and robust. They had listened to the litany of risks but had at some level not wanted to credit them. The video of it all ran unbidden in my head several times each day for the next several weeks, less often over the next year or so.

We neurosurgeons are caricatured as filled with conceit, short on empathy. And there's truth in that cartoon. But hubris is tough to maintain while completing and signing your patient's death certificate. It erodes as the Jane Does grow in number, collapses in the private cemetery of unwelcome memories.

Although we had met the moment and had done our best work, the illness had been too much for us. The malpractice suit that followed was not entirely a surprise. This was a law student after all. His lawyers predicted a bright future for him and insisted that we were too inexperienced to have tackled such a rare and dangerous problem, that we should have put him on a plane to London, Ontario. Our defense was strong. Dr. Wilson would act as our expert, vouch for our skills, and emphasize the danger of this aneurysm regardless of who managed it, would detail the risks of re-rupture with pressurized airplane travel. But our insurance company feared going to trial against the ghost of such an attractive plaintiff. The suit settled for what they considered a small sum, and no more basilar aneurysms went to a Topeka OR. Ironically, as interventional radiology has advanced, these cases are seldom treated surgically anywhere today.

I've written mostly about intracranial surgery, but it represented only about one-third of our practice. Spine trouble was far more common in our eastern Kansas demographic. About once a month I'd open my exam room door to see someone with a ruptured lumbar disc and enter to find the exam table empty, my new patient curled on the floor. "The pain's not so bad down here," was the common refrain. These folks said nothing about their back but complained of terrific sciatic leg pain. Scans showed dramatic nerve compression, the squashed nerve root often invisible, obscured completely by fragments of ruptured disc (the spongy shock absorber between the bones of the spine). Their leg was often disabled by loss of power and sensation, but they sometimes didn't recognize their deficit in the face of such pain.

Their surgical procedure was common, but to label it routine would be cavalier. The incision at the midline of the lower back was about two inches long, the dissection down to the spine compulsively midline to minimize bleeding and postop pain, sweeping muscles back away from bone. A bit of bone from two adjacent vertebrae would be removed, enough to admit the tip of my ring finger. At the bottom of that bony opening I'd find the blue-gray dura and its lateral edge, then the origin of the compressed nerve root as it began its path between those two vertebrae. Its course then would take it beyond the surgical field deep into the buttock where it would join three of its neighbors to form the sciatic nerve. As the compression was relieved, the two centimeters of exposed root would typically double in size, more purple than its usual creamy gray. Removal of the disc fragments, looking and feeling for all the world like morsels of crabmeat, would allow the newly swollen root to relax and to pulse with each heartbeat and click of anesthesia's ventilator.

These folks were delighted even in the recovery room, sometimes eager to go home later in the day. Word of such dramatic success would spread quickly in our little town. The feeling of triumph was seductive, tempting a surgeon to bend the rules, to intervene when not all criteria were fully met. I thought back to those Bay Area surgeons who did too much.

Low back pain is endemic in America and so has attracted many sketchy, skillfully-marketed treatments. Because the pain so often resolves spontaneously, those treatments seem to "work"—and do create serious profit. Lasers caught Kansans' imagination in those days. My San Francisco experience with excessive spine surgery had helped draw me to Topeka, and we were consistently conservative in our patient selection, widely known not to be "knife happy." But radicular limb pain is so intense and its surgical relief so dramatic that our reputation grew, coming gradually to rest on a growing collection of relieved citizens—Goodyear tire builders, schoolteachers, beauticians, cops.

Seeing patients and their families at the drug store or the multiplex discouraged flamboyant surgical behavior. But as diagnostic imaging became more sophisticated, patients and their doctors were often tempted to conflate structural findings on an MRI with clinical complaints, magically equating structure with function. Operations based on that temptation usually fail or succeed only by accident. Spinal function (and dysfunction) is very much a movie, not fully captured by a static image, however precise. A careful history and exam is much cheaper and far more valuable for diagnosis. And ironically, spinal surgery is often more effective for limb symptoms than for spinal pain.

Not every case hovered between life and death. But each new

patient carried with them into the exam room a twinge of fear, a fear that stopped their ears. I would see many patients each day. Those folks would see a neurosurgeon once in their lifetime, if they were fortunate. No escaping their disquiet.

So, job one became reassurance as a hearing aid—humor, slow conversation in short English words. No fancy language. These people were disarmed, short of clothing and surgical expertise. I made certain to wear a necktie every day. Partly as ancient armor, partly as male plumage, partly as reassurance—that I took them and their visit seriously. To hear their own voice tell their story and to watch me write it down gave them much needed agency, balanced the scales a bit. My first question always invited them to talk for a minute or two, a surprisingly long time for me to sit still and hold my tongue.

I learned to read them as we spoke—a new furrow on the forehead, a quick look toward a spouse, a restless twitch of the legs, pale knuckles deforming a handbag strap. All suggested that I slow the conversation. Their body language was always eloquent, but my comprehension, my fluency, came only with time and practice. I had been raised to be exquisitely sensitive to others' fear and anger, a skill at first for survival, a skill now fundamental to empathic bedside manner. I paid undivided attention in those little rooms. But the encounters, four in a typical day, wore me out.

We were a monopoly in Northeastern Kansas, so we had the power to practice conservatively, the power to influence the conditions of our work—which nurses we worked with, which overpriced equipment the hospitals might buy. We chose to balance that power with a responsibility to take all comers, insured or not, to see ourselves as something of a public good, a kind of surgical utility. The decision brought us a rising tide of excruciating encounters.

A short order cook came to the office in those years after having had a seizure. The ER had done a CT scan and referred him for treatment. With him were his cheerful young wife and rambunctious two-year-old son. The scan showed a large malignant tumor, foretelling a swift but likely painless death. Short order cooks usually weren't offered health insurance. He was no exception. They'd just moved into a starter home.

I knew well how to deliver bad medical news, but these financial catastrophes were beyond my skills, left me heartsick. Our tiny rooms already overflowed with anguish. We waived our fees, but bills from anesthesia, pathology, operating room, recovery room et al., were more than enough to swallow their house, exile the boy to distant relatives, and destroy their marriage. This horror had no author, was of course no one's fault. No one to blame. Our institutions could simply be cruel, as my ancestors had known for lifetimes. There was no villain in this tale, but the deck was thoroughly stacked. I became an early fan of national health insurance.

We had our triumphs and our catastrophes, but my memory is far from even-handed. I recall my failures with brilliant clarity because I was taught that the best doctors make no errors and that I was exactly as good as my last result.

A young woman survived a jump from the Golden Gate Bridge in 1974 and arrived at San Francisco General in cardiac arrest. When I became her intern on the trauma service, she'd been in the ICU for three months and had suffered every post-traumatic complication known to the house staff. She hadn't wakened and had been pulled from death every few days with aggressive resuscitation. She died during my last week on that service, and I organized her volumes of clinical records so that our chief resident could present her case to the senior faculty at mortality and morbidity rounds. He detailed her saga and awaited the professors' comments.

The chairman of the department of surgery gave him a level look, then asked whether her death had been a result of "an error in technique or an error in judgment." His message, explicit in that moment but conveyed wordlessly each day, was that we brilliant, tireless physicians could push death away, maintain it perpetually at arm's length, always more an option than a necessity. So, we could sometimes be good enough, but competence was forever transient.

STEEP

This gorge had no exit, the mountain no summit. His pedagogy made for good theater and fixed us in a state of fear, but over time it eroded honesty, tempting us all to advertise success and bury error. His lesson took years to unlearn.

The OR held images of the sublime. Each recalled several hours well spent. The anatomical neighborhoods of the nervous system manifest who we humans are and some of what we can do. So much function in so little space is cause for awe. But even more than these visits to God's country, I treasured bearing witness to my fellow Kansans inhabiting the peaks and valleys of their own lives. Many eminent surgeons care for a parade of strangers—I worked where most everyone knew my name or knew someone who did. The almost-blind woman reading the comics the day after removal of her pituitary tumor, the old man enjoying normal sphincter function and sexual life after decompression of the nerves of his lower spine. The inexplicable courage of so many patients and families to meet the worst news they could receive. They all gave this young man a priceless and intimate education. I was helpful on my good days, did my share of good turns. I had the experience and hope I didn't miss too much of its meaning.

A ranching family from near Matfield Green, a small community almost 100 miles south of Topeka, brought their matriarch to see me in 1998 about a serious problem. Three generations packed our waiting room for what under other circumstances might have been a family reunion. She was the family's anchor, also the ranch's accountant and personnel manager. The problem was that she had lost her mind, the hope that I might help her retrieve it. She was about 60, her husband a taciturn block of muscle in faded Dickie bib overalls, no stranger to hard work but now very much at sea. Their two sons sported alligator boots and saucer-sized silver belt buckles emblematic of rodeo success, but their hands were as hard as his. As we greeted, they showed restraint. Their hands could easily have fractured mine.

Her history was not unusual. Several years before she had complained of loss of smell, had gradually lost her taste for food and her knack in the kitchen. Her daughters had begun cooking for the family and staff. Next, she seemed to withdraw, increasingly abrupt and profane. Personal hygiene declined, and most recently she had been unable to reconcile the ranch's books. She had become a different person.

The presumptive diagnosis had been Alzheimer's disease, her MRI done in part to placate her family, almost an afterthought. Instead, it gave dramatic reason for her decline: a tumor arising directly behind the center of her forehead, flattening both waterlogged frontal lobes against the inner skull, bright as a headlight on the enhanced scan sequences and nearly the size of a navel orange.

As I put the scans up onto the exam room view boxes, they stole the show. Her family was drawn to the magical technology, chattering over this exquisite anatomical demonstration of a human brain. I struggled for half a minute to get anyone's attention. This was surely a benign tumor, a meningioma, which had developed over many years, gradually corroding personality and cognition. She was awake but absent and flat, hastily buffed for the trip to the big city, her steel gray hair clearly in need of a trim. Her fingernails had escaped her family's attention. Her forearms were an anatomical demonstration, each muscle and tendon testifying to decades of toil. I found no excess body fat.

This was the sort of case neurosurgeons covet. A chance to bring a cure, a recovery of mind and self. A colleague once described what we do as playing in the World Series every day. In a few days she and I might be deep into extra innings of game 7. My feelings were mixed, though, because I'd really need my support hose. This would take all day. And the most dangerous moments would come several hours in, when the back of the tumor came away from the structures behind it—major arteries, cranial nerves, superior brainstem. Its posterior capsule would either be stuck to those structures or not, the risk of dissection low or high. No way to predict. I was suddenly tired just looking at the scan and regretted I had no residents to help open and close this monster.

Much good-natured family jostling and fussy whispering

greeted the scans displayed on those view boxes. I was enlisted to answer a flood of insightful questions about how magnetic fields worked to create these arresting images, about how Mom could have lived harboring such a big tumor, and of course about what could be done. Theirs was a large ranch. They could have gone anywhere for care. But they ran down a roster of people I'd seen over almost 20 years as their reason to be in Topeka that day. I struggled to remember most of the names. Many were managers or laborers at the Iowa Beef plant in Emporia.

Surely this little room was my turf, yet these ranchers were examining me. I had to reclaim a slice of it by gently evicting one from my exam room stool so I could sit down. We were foreign to each other, their Kansas roots more than a century deeper than mine. I'd come to Topeka two decades earlier as something of an internally displaced person, chafing at tribal loyalties. But now I felt fitted to the moment, at peace with their scrutiny and at ease with my past.

The younger generation, 30-somethings, were intensely curious about mechanics, about the nuts and bolts of the operation itself. So. This tumor arises not from the brain itself but from the meninges, the membranes that surround it. When the cells of these meninges become inflamed, a patient is said to have meningitis. And when they give rise to a tumor it's known as a meningioma. The surgeon needs to remove the entire bone of the forehead to gain access to this site but is expected to leave the patient cosmetically unchanged after surgery. The incision to do that is a very long inverted letter U, extending like a bucket handle from just in front of one ear, running just behind the hairline over the top of the head to the equivalent spot just in front of the opposite ear. The scalp is folded down over the nose and the frontal bone of the forehead removed as a single block and put into antiseptic. The dura, the outer layer of the meninges, is opened and then—well, this tumor would not be hard to find.

Tumors in this spot get their blood supply from below, from the base of the skull, so working from the bottom first would minimize blood loss and shorten our day. Also, it would be important to create working space from within the tumor as long as we could. To gut it while minimizing contact with the distressed and fragile frontal lobes on either side. Nothing vital to neurologic function would be found inside this tumor, only at its capsule.

Their questions were blunt. They understood risk, lived daily with life and death. They were more than ready to learn and quantify the various minor and major hazards. But I suspect that they had decided to go forward in Topeka before we'd met and were using our conversation to take my measure.

Incision came at 8 a.m. I had expert help from our scrub nurse, Lil Thompson. Her skill flowed as much from knowing me and the particular rhythm of this operation as from her knowledge of the gleaming thicket of instruments on her Mayo stand and back table. Many surgeons, myself included, lose the faculty of speech under extreme stress. To receive the right instrument wordlessly into your hand in the proper position of function at that instant makes a real difference for the patient.

I was grateful to get lunch relief from Arjunan, my partner. Circulating nurses and anesthesia changed shifts at about 3 p.m., just as I was appreciating the fact that the posterior capsule of this tumor would dissect away easily from the vital territory behind it. The gods were smiling, and my legs were deeply grateful.

With the tumor gone, I took a long look down the barrels of the microscope at the base of the brain, to revel in the miraculous. I'd seen this anatomy many times, but its magic simply would not fade. I surveyed a sacred landscape—the major arteries and optic nerves in the foreground, the pituitary and brainstem in the distance. The colors ranging from calm cream to magenta to fiery red, the structures dull or gleaming in their turn. This task had tested my mastery, had demanded hours of undivided attention, and had carried potent meaning. We reached the recovery room at about 4:30.

She did well, well enough to resume her position in the family and in the business. And to be her old self in her husband's eyes. As good as it gets. The anatomy was magical, but the entire encounter sticks in memory. For many years, each time I had knocked on an exam room door to meet a new patient, I held in mind the shape of a perfect encounter. Insightful history with no misdirected questions, focused examination guided by that history. Patient's questions addressed; fears assuaged. And perfection in the OR had its own image. No unnecessary moves, no collateral injury, minimal blood loss. A violent event clothed in delicacy and infused with practiced grace. A peak moment. Her case brought me closer to that standard than I'd ever been.

She returned to the office six weeks after discharge with only her husband, this visit far less dramatic than her first. She was reserved and watchful, the lenses of her pearl-gray reading glasses polished to perfect clarity, her fingernails rehabilitated, her new gray wig battened down. She was once more an accountant and a manager. He wore the same overalls and battered boots. She did complain that the scalp behind her incision was numb, and I assured her normal sensation would return over the next several months. She scanned the walls of my tiny exam room, decorated with the usual diplomas and licenses. She thanked me for my efforts, then reminded her husband that she'd never been in this room. He opened his mouth to argue, his jaw falling for an instant. He was astonished by this erasure of memory. I was not.

As we stood to say goodbye, I casually asked about life in Matfield Green and promptly unleashed a river of words from this laconic man. He basked in the doctor's attention, discoursing on long-range weather forecasting models and the machinations of the Chicago futures market. He rhapsodized about the beauty of his land, riffed in detail and at length on the too-generous price supports his Argentinian competitors received.

After a couple of minutes my patient began to glance from her watch to her husband with a mix of irritation and alarm. She fingered the straps of her purse, seemingly an unfamiliar accessory. Finally, she stood and announced their departure, smiling and gently pulling him from the room by a strap of his overalls. "Harold, this man has work to do—and so do we," she said. I was actually delighted at his tutorial and relieved to keep no one waiting. She was my day's last patient. I'd often been glad to teach in that little room and now was glad to learn.

Three days had passed for my Aryan motorcyclist. We had reduced the pressure in his brain, his labs looked good. His scalp wounds were closed, his road rash scrubbed up. We had unleashed the full bore of high-tech medicine on his body, but he would not waken. I had registered the ink, the bold black block letters on his chest at our first meeting but made no pause in the work, felt an instant of sadness but no fear, and so no anger. The clinical reflexes and ancestral stoicism that had long governed me now blessed him, converting provocation to wallpaper. And of course, I knew well that more than a few of my fellow Kansans carried the same tattoo stenciled deep within their minds.

This moment of equanimity was frail and had cost a lot, but I would give my best effort and so could relax with whatever came next. These skirmishes, these affronts to our humanity, actually come every day, though seldom so dramatically. They aren't unique to emergency rooms and don't limit themselves to the writers of books. They play out for all of us before the smallest of audiences. They arrive by stealth and by surprise. The ICU nurses and I persisted.

He was spared exploratory surgery that first night by an emergency CT that showed an angry swollen cerebral landscape much like that of Jane Doe decades earlier. He had only one visitor during his weeks in the hospital, a ghostly young woman who appeared in the early hours of one morning, did not share her name and did not return. Our social workers scoured their databases but unearthed no family. His solitary struggle and persistent coma complicated our decision making—how aggressively to treat his complications, his sepsis and respiratory distress. He received cutting edge care and did not die quickly but vegetated for nearly a year in a local nursing home.

STEEP

Several years later I saw a 20-year-old kid unconscious after a gunshot wound. The entrance wound at the back of his head showed powder burns and the larger exit wound in his forehead oozed a bit of frontal lobe with each sigh of the ventilator. An assassination. Patients typically don't survive this injury, and he wouldn't be an exception. As a young surgeon I'd operated aggressively on many people unlikely to recover their selves, or to recover at all. I'd brought that happy ferocity from my training, in part because I was forever moving to the next rotation, never seeing the ultimate outcomes of my heroic efforts. But being embedded in a community meant confronting long term results. And a few visits to the nursing homes of Topeka tempered my zeal. I knew this story and my role all too well.

The complexity that night wasn't the patient's injury, a common tragedy leavened by organ donation, if at all. He wasn't alone in his tiny walled ER cubicle. He shared it with five of his friends, all dressed in identical shades of red and black. How they'd all reached that space I don't know. Maybe hospital security had been between shifts. I found myself nudging between them, excusing myself to do my work. They were large, made larger by their blackness and by the menace that hung in the air. They showed no grief, no anger, only those flat eyes Dad had cautioned me about. I'd trekked a long way from that warning in Roxbury so many years before. And I believe now that their eyes conveyed distance more than vacancy or anger that night. A vast space, silently voicing the idea that we definitely are not all in this together.

But the practical lesson from training was to finish my exam at the patient's feet and say nothing until I was between his family and the door. I explained from the foot of the bed how severe his injury was, that I couldn't find any evidence of brain activity on my bedside exam, that we'd do an EEG to look for signs of brain life—or death. Their only question, repeated three times, was how soon I would be waking their friend up. I worked to wish them all well, though I knew their friend's future as well as I knew my name.

Finally, a young man headed to the OR after a car wreck. I spoke with his large, frantic family in the pre-op holding area, outlining what I planned to do, along with the risks, benefits and alternatives—a standard informed consent talk. In these situations, families and surgeons both face serious obstacles. The family must adapt quickly, must understand and act on the reality that their member, recently healthy, is now desperately ill, and perhaps trust an absolute stranger who suddenly holds a position of unique importance. The doctor does well to recognize their struggle and work to establish something like instant intimacy.

That day's lesson from training was to identify the family's linchpin and address every word to her. Her, because that linchpin was often an older woman. I had aimed my words well. The patient's grandmother was able to restrain his estranged Dad after he had grabbed my shirt and screamed into my face not to fuck up—by smacking him in the head with her purse, sending him stumbling back into a nurse's arms.

Yes. Such training is useful, necessary—but insufficient. Encounters like these three invited me to move past competence. Welcoming these wounded souls, these strangers, these ancestral enemies as fellow travelers sounded simple but carried near infinite cost. I couldn't possibly succeed, could aim only to fail better each day. The effort was what mattered. The rest was not my business.

And yet. The effort had its effect, the action its result. Karma became real. As the years and the cases flew by, my hair whitened and my reputation for compassion grew. That word's Latin origin means "suffering with." Some in the doctors' lounge shamed their patients' ignorance or weight or smell. A few of those unwashed souls saw me for second opinions and, in tears or in rage, told of being ridiculed face to face. I could guess what mix of fear and ignorance colonized these doctors' minds. My dark skin had inoculated me against this flavor of cruelty, had willed me an outsider's perspective, a kind of cultural leprosy—a profoundly mixed blessing. On my good days I could retrieve that life at the margins, could excavate that history and change places with the folks on those exam tables. Could make care for the patient drive the care of the patient.

A gracious home, a beautiful spouse, our boys at the threshold of adolescence. We were building a life in this eastern corner of the Great Plains. But I took too little note of Mary's parents' decline and their move to Topeka. They'd become shadows of themselves, facing depression and electroshock therapy, hydrocephalus and subdural hematomas. The Kafkaesque jousts with Medicare, the negotiations with assisted living, and the unending parade of appointments swallowed Mary's attention and stole something from her life's prime. And now I was back on every-other-night call for both ERs as the boys moved into the trials of their teenage years.

As we recruited a third partner, we were quickly reminded that aspiring neurosurgeons were seldom drawn to towns like Topeka. Our hopes rocketed when our recruiter sent us an unbelievable resume. Stephen Dell, brother to computer magnate Michael, wanted to look at our practice. He boasted credentials from several major medical centers and glowing letters of recommendation from well-known professors. We quickly arranged a visit and forwarded him details of our situation. We welcomed him to Topeka, putting the best face on ourselves and our little town. I, of course, had made an unexpected choice in coming to Kansas but now struggled to fathom his motivations. He was polite and friendly, although he struck a false note in our kitchen when he pointedly asked how a busy neurosurgeon could live in such a modest home. After he'd left to think over our offer, I noticed that he'd spent a short time at Cornell University Medical Center. Neurosurgery is a very small band, and I knew someone who'd overlapped his time there. That someone was a friend, by then the chairman of neurosurgery at the University of Michigan. I called and asked about Dr. Dell. He replied, "Craig, listen closely. Do not recruit him. Do not return his calls. Do not answer his letters. Have nothing to do with him. Am I clear?" I was certainly unhappy but by no means confused. I'd never had such unvarnished advice, couldn't even voice a reply. We withdrew our offer with serious reluctance.

Six months later on a Sunday evening, Arjunan phoned to insist that we quickly turn on *60 Minutes* to see their expose on Dr. Dell, revealed as hopping from one practice to the next, always one step ahead of state licensing boards. Our desperation had nearly undone us. Several months later we were lucky to find John Ebeling, a fine surgeon and avid hunter, a clear and present danger to Kansas' turkey population. He knew the hills of eastern Kansas well and I suspect that he actually found us, attracted both to the practice and the game.

15 nights per month tethered to the local ERs again became 10. Travel became more possible, sometimes to glamorous cities for neurosurgical meetings. This one, in LA, began with a lavish cocktail reception at Disneyland. I had taken a run that smoggy afternoon and began to wheeze as we socialized. My asthma had been episodic over many years. Most recently, though, I'd been well. I had perfect faith in my rescue inhaler and imagined my illness was well controlled, suffering that evening from hypoxia aggravated by egotism. Mary saved me, dragging me into a cab for the Cedars Sinai Hospital ER. I don't remember the cab ride but do recall her fear, voiced to me as exasperation. I imagined that working just a bit harder would move enough air to get me well. Too little oxygen or too little imagination to be afraid. In the ER my blood pressure was through the roof and my oxygen levels through the floor. The IV saline was chilly and the nasal oxygen welcome. And those hours of IV steroids and breathing treatments rebooted my life.

The boys played sports, of course. I marveled at their grace. Still do. They learned about team play and about winning and losing. Mary rescued us all from the temptations of overdressed, overtraveled, overcoached competition. She saw clearly the trials of interstate travel for her kids and was free from the sports mania so commonly tied to the Y chromosome. But indoor soccer resurrected my past on one winter afternoon.

Zack's middle school team was to travel to Kansas City for a match. The stated goal was to maintain fitness, but this was definitely a step up in competition for our small-town squad. The

STEEP

KC team's "home field" was a gymnasium floor covered with astroturf, far smaller than a standard pitch. The ball could be played off the walls and so couldn't go out of bounds, making play continuous. Our opponents' flashy uniforms and exotic warm up routine reinforced our psychological disadvantage.

This indoor game was very much a contact sport, more hockey than soccer, and our boys were seriously overmatched. We parents looked on from an elevated running track converted into an observation deck, the home team's folks giddy with delight at the ongoing rout. Viewing space at the railing was limited. I stepped up when one of the local dads walked away. He wore a heavy canvas shirt and carried a whiff of onion rings. Gray eyes were lodged deep in a puffy face. He soon returned, poked my left shoulder and demanded that I leave "his" spot. I gripped the railing in some version of shock, unable to speak. He grabbed my left wrist.

To blink requires about 0.2 seconds—too little time to fit a thought between stimulus and response. In that interval I pivoted left, locked onto his belt with my free right hand, and whirled to toss him over the railing to the pitch 40 feet below. He was short and stout, at least 180 pounds. I lifted him with ridiculous ease but was instantly bearhugged by the father of our team's star player. He aborted my crime of passion, saved the would-be murderer along with the victim. I'd been scaling sheer walls for years, imagining that I could transcend my past, but in this instant, I was falling free into a pit of stifling heat and scarce air—into my personal hell on earth. My ancestors screamed wordless volumes of shame and rage in those 0.2 seconds.

We warring dads backed away from each other without a word and I stalked out of the gym to cool off in the cold, watching exhaled water vapor leave my lungs, uncomfortably aware of my temporal arteries hammering against the lining of my black wool knit cap. I was unable to think for several minutes and unsettled for days. I had grown up decades before, aiming for a simpler version of fatherhood now misplaced in time. I might as well have been a knight errant charging windmills.

Zack rode home in the backseat of our van, happily plugged into his music, quickly putting the loss behind him, unaware of the drama above his head on the running track. Reason, as much as clothing, expertise, and credentials had long served as armor in my jousts with a hostile world. How could it all be so instantly undone? "I think, therefore I am," wrote Descartes. But he was seriously mistaken. The great majority of our brain's mass has no role, no interest in thought. We are primates. Advanced, perhaps rising, but primates. In that blind moment I was founded in ancient impulse, not in thought. I was leading the life of a volatile stranger.

-7-
TWILIGHT OF EXPERTISE

I was in particularly good spirits on a Sunday morning in 1985, free from my beeper, enjoying good coffee and a serene family moment. The ring of our doorbell revealed a pleasant, portly middle-aged man in a too-tight dark suit. He smiled, asked my name, then handed me a subpoena naming me a defendant in a malpractice suit demanding 40 million dollars. My coffee went cold. The morning disappeared. And the ensuing ordeal commandeered my mind for the next 18 months.

I struggled even to recognize the plaintiff's name but soon learned that he'd been an intoxicated young soldier who had wrecked his new Ford Cobra GT against a bridge abutment on I-70 two years before. He'd suffered multiple significant injuries, but his head trauma had anointed me his attending physician. We had transferred him to a VA hospital in Houston after about a week, still deeply comatose but recovering from his femur fracture, torn spleen and flail chest. His ultimate outcome was spectacular, far better than statistically predicted. He had recovered normal cognition and mobility but had been left hoarse. And we in Topeka had failed to recognize his fractured larynx.

This suit was remarkable for several reasons. First, these fractures typically present with complaints of hoarseness, but recognizing a husky voice in a comatose, ventilated patient would have been a challenge. Second, although we'd failed to diagnose the fracture we had treated it properly by coincidence. The tube in his windpipe was actually a standard treatment for his fracture, and he'd been intubated throughout his time in Topeka for his chest and brain injuries. Third, some hoarseness was likely after any laryngeal fracture, regardless of how it had been treated. Finally, his dad was wealthy enough to pay his son's lawyers by the hour rather than on contingency, ensuring near-endless litigation.

After much pretrial legal skirmishing, our defense swallowed 10 days in federal court. I'd been forged for this kind of combat since childhood, of course. My enemies were in plain sight. I understood I was very much the visiting team on the witness stand and became a vanishingly-small though unfailingly-gracious target of cross examination. Mom would have admired the exquisite courtesy that cloaked my venom.

The jury awarded my opponent zero dollars. But victory was expensive. The trek corroded my outlook, converted each new patient into a potential litigant, each clinical note into a grotesquely enlarged courtroom exhibit. I emerged harder, more heavily armored, more deeply bunkered. The ordeal was a body blow to a kid whose identity was yoked to his competence. And the armor weighed a lot—exactly as much as the dark husky boy with the clubbed foot required.

Malpractice litigation has never aspired to improve medical practice, but rather to compensate the victims of medical error. And that it does poorly. Our mistakes harming the old and the poor yield many fewer dollars for the litigators than those harming the young and well paid, and so are less often pursued. Contingency arrangements pay the lawyer almost as well as the victim, and the glacial pace of the process erodes what relief ultimately arrives. Our care would improve if state licensing boards had real authority to restrict clinical privileges and to publicize errors as the invaluable learning tools they are. And no-fault compensation to victims would serve everyone better.

I made dozens of decisions each day in my 25 years of practice. What to do, to not do. Who came first, who last. A torrent of judgments, many trivial, some not. I was sued nine times in those years, a number a bit below the national average for neurosurgeons. Three were justified, three frivolous, and three debatable. What's not debatable is that I made far more than nine errors over those 25 years —most inconsequential, a few deadly. The worst still come to mind uninvited. Doctors are quick to decry the costs of malpractice insurance coverage, and it was always our biggest expense, about a thousand dollars per week per surgeon. But more painful for me was the recurring legal combat that gradually pulled a creeping tide of cynicism into my mind. Navigating an adversarial world was my birthright. But now the ascent had squeezed me into a blind cul-de-sac. I wondered how I might change the script of this unhappy drama.

After three astonishing weeks of family vacation in India in 1999 we returned to our sedate hometown. I was reluctant but ready to repay my partners and absorb a siege of night call. Each visit to those ERs now brought fresh evidence that life is short, evidence instantly available to any physician with eyes to see. We're told that time is money, but that's mercantile fiction. Time counts far more — a cliche easy to recite but hard to reify. I saw ever more advanced technology overapplied and heavily reimbursed, the cost routinely dwarfing the benefit. Decades of medical miracles on TV dramas and a flood of prime-time drug ads had vaulted public expectations far beyond clinical reality. Flickering images that starred the young and the telegenic, the sick nowhere to be found.

We all are reaching for reassurance in this brave new secular world — the certainties of Sunday mornings and church clothes gone with *On the Origin of Species*. But our fear of death hasn't disappeared and won't any time soon. We reach for salvation now from wellness gurus, from influencers, from remote autocrats. I saw many folks in their moment of terror when neurosurgeons ranked high on that list of saviors. Their eyes saw a shaman, idolized me along with the technology I wielded. And when those idols fail, their devotees are left to wander in a sterile wilderness.

More of these ER disasters seemed self-inflicted now, and I was less quick to recover for the next day's elective surgery than I'd been a few years before. Too many of these Kansans became organ donors, enough that I continued to win awards from the Midwest Organ Bank. Great for the recipients, dubious for me. The local hospitals were at war, the air increasingly mercenary. Dueling TV ads promoted exclusive, value-added services. To win admitting privileges at one meant exile from the other. The Hatfields and McCoys had traded in their shotguns for MRI scanners and marketing firms.

I had learned to practice in a time before electronic medical records, hospitalists, and intensivists. My bedside skills were losing value, and I didn't warm to my new work of data entry. The computer terminal and its electronic medical record took up precious headspace and square footage in my crowded exam room—and failed to read my patients' unspoken messages. My attention was easily fractured, my multitasking barely mediocre.

Meanwhile, we had lived well but carefully. In some years we'd managed to honor the memory of Corey Road and save a third of our income, disloyal behavior in an American culture of perpetual acquisition. At each quarterly meeting our financial planners would gently remind us that I could stop operating if I chose, that their game of buy and sell was over, that we had won. But I was fixed in disbelief, rooted in my inherited faith that the very notion of enough money was oxymoronic fiction.

I had often listened to grand words from the pulpit about a rich man's road to heaven being as broad as a camel's path through a needle's eye. Now I wondered whether his obstacle wasn't so much net worth as a deficit of attention, the excessive headroom taken and held by his fear of scarcity, or worse. I was clinging to identity too, taking refuge in expertise, though by now the work was feeling all too familiar.

These ruminations were too much for Dad. He asked with a mix of anxiety and irritation how he could brag to his friends if I retired. He needed a ten-minute answer or none at all. I'd made a steep climb from the warren of Corey Road, had paid a high price for this whiff of freedom. I just shook my head in wonder and hugged his rock-hard barrel chest for a long moment. My technical skills and my reputation were peaking. My ancestors chanted that I hadn't done enough, or well enough. But I really had done a great deal, and after 25 years, enough was finally enough. Enough clipped aneurysms and broken necks. Enough brain tumors. Enough short nights and mayhem. And enough tears.

On January 1, 2003, I left surgical practice, testing the value of time over money. This was no thought experiment. I'd spent almost 30 years in operating rooms, but believed that there was life beyond those gleaming, sterile walls. Like most surgical subspecialists, I knew a great deal about not much, had become a virtuoso short on repertoire. Life as an expert had grown comfortable, its dance too easily predicted. My world was small and shrinking as I grew old.

The work had rewarded my family and my town. It had rewarded me in many ways. My patients benefited from my experience of thousands of cases. But the liquid fuel of centuries of ancestral tears powering this human missile had run low, and to leave the OR was to test history's power head-on and in real time. Did Baldwin have it right? Was my past so indelibly tattooed within me? Leaving carried risk but also opened a path away from assigned identity, a chance for some measure of liberation. I was 54 years old, and in this end could be my beginning.

I'd long been living too much in the minds of strangers, a proxy for ancient grievance. My life had been driven, coherent, short on humor and surprise. Now the missile had reached its target, gliding into retirement on fumes. What next? Could I redirect this stealth weapon, shed a layer or two of armor? Could I retire my ancestral debt? Could I recast the missile as a spade—unearth my past and prefigure a future in some wider world? Or would I detonate and chase my tail into senescence?

The unmapped journey would begin in midlife, just as I had "arrived." I had given the hospitals and my partners a year's notice to replace me, but corporate distrust aggravated the challenge of recruiting. Three years of political intrigue followed—many candidates, many recruiting visits, many contract squabbles. By 2006 the hospitals had spent heavily to establish entirely separate neurosurgical practices, doubling the number of surgeons in town to six.

My first conscious action of 1/1/2003 was to unplug our

bedroom phone, unleashing weeks of stunningly vivid dreams. What I'd accepted for decades as sleep had actually been a chronic semi-waking state. How I had roused to do a trying job for those many years remains a mystery. But now I was more awake than I'd been in decades, inching away from the gnawing fear that had come with each ring of that telephone, the fear that I might do some ill soul serious harm.

On January 2, I started training for the Mothers' Day marathon in Lincoln, Nebraska. It was now or never for these asthmatic lungs. My body very much wanted to remain horizontal under warm down blankets in the blackness of those winter mornings. My first few steps each day came with serious ambivalence, and the training was far more difficult than the race. I questioned my sanity on a few of those predawn expeditions through Topeka's vacant streets. But I knew plenty about running. I'd been chasing one medal or another for longer than I could remember.

The big day featured a persistent light rain and a long gentle climb at mile 21. My soaked, leaden feet went the distance, and I finished upright and running but failed to recognize Mary as she cheered me on through the last 100 meters of the four-hour-and-12-minute ordeal. My body had been recreated and the experience had asked pointed questions of my mind. I'd answered well but wondered whether I'd been chasing Dr. Wilson and his Boston Marathon bib all along. More tangled motives—more running, climbing. But I did know on that drizzly day that I'd answered well enough, had done well enough for once, whatever my ancestors' laments. DuBois' Talented Tenth made space for an aging jock. And I still do run (actually shuffle) a few miles each week to help maintain this exquisite machine I occupy.

I had silenced my beeper. We could go now, go to a few of those lands I'd imagined through the haze of cigar smoke in that Harvard Square newsstand. Take ourselves from our home on the range out onto the road. See more of Kansas. My mind could gradually, fitfully, make space for the present, hear its shouts and, with practice, its whispers—look less to the future which had enticed for so long.

I first learned of Chartres Cathedral in 1990 from Joseph Campbell. *The Power of Myth*, a written conversation between him and Bill Moyers, held an honored spot on my nightstand for years. We'd long itched to visit and in 2017 took the one-hour train ride south from Paris to reach it. It had begun as a country church. But the iconic gothic architecture was the stuff of textbooks, and the building embodied a faith both wide and deep. Its air was cool, old, carrying the memory of uncounted candles. There was room for many to belong in this 1,200-year-old space. The power of belief was everywhere. The windows, visual instruction for medieval peasants, spoke eloquently to me in the present tense. Generations had ended their climb of faith here. The cobalt blue foretold the face of heaven. I wielded my cell phone camera with unpracticed enthusiasm. We didn't face big crowds that day, but the building would easily have withstood a small army of visitors. The spiritual space was immense.

We learned that at the approach of the German army in 1940, the local bishop had recruited a group of boys too young to fight and had tasked them with removing each piece of glass for cataloging and burial. Each window was then reconstructed, beginning in 1946. I had been overpowered in larger, more famous sanctuaries, but felt more at peace here. We stayed that night in an elegant Best Western hotel two blocks away, our window looking out on the cathedral and fixing it in memory.

A few days later we visited Saint Chappelle in Paris. Like many other landmarks, it was under Islamist threat. The two guards on duty at the entrance were active-duty military but they were also chatty teenage girls, makeup and body armor carefully applied, assault rifles casually at the ready, cradled in manicured hands— manifesting some uniquely French response to terrorism. This aging child soldier could have used some of their laughter on Corey Road. This world was more complex, more beautiful than I'd dreamed. I couldn't resist asking for a photo. They merrily agreed and Mary captured a digital image of the unlikely trio.

By 2006 I was restless to be more than a retired doctor, itching for a new climb. I knew something about health care and felt pulled to public service. Governor Kathleen Sebelius asked that I be the medical advisor to her new Kansas Health Policy Authority. I quickly learned from my boss that healthcare was far from the agency's primary mission. Head count, office space, budget, and access to the governor were the coins of this realm. I wrote a couple of reasonable position papers on the meaning of quality in medicine but was mostly a poor fit in an agency promptly disbanded by Kathleen's successor. I chafed in the bureaucracy and craved instant recognition, no surprise for this retired surgeon. An op-ed on healthcare I wrote for our local paper was faulted. I'd written as a private citizen, promoting simplicity in insurance and closer attention to public health. My ideas were hardly radical but had emerged unexpectedly from the middle of the Authority's org chart. I was cautioned that my role didn't allow for a private voice—and took the opportunity to resign. I had failed as a team player, or had joined the wrong team. Squeezed between history and misplaced ambition, I had chosen to ascend the wrong ladder, a soloist in search of an audience.

I began volunteering in 2004 at the Marian Clinic, a service for the working uninsured. A few folks there were anxious to get narcotics or disability income, but most were solid citizens, and all were resourceful — long on savvy and short of luck. They welcomed my attention. I could sometimes see them grow straighter and taller in front of my eyes. And in 2009 my former partners asked me to do a kind of office triage, to take a part-time role seeing people unlikely to benefit from surgery, allowing them to see obvious surgical candidates more promptly. I relished the lost arts of taking a good history and doing a thorough exam. I was no longer the surgeon for these folks, no longer top gun. But my experience had value.

Teaching these anxious people something about their illness reliably gave them a measure of power over it. Freedom, really. And everyone loves to be heard, especially by a neurosurgeon.

But my political itch persisted, born of an old dissonance. We on Corey Road had been highly informed and totally impotent, venerating public figures while dismissing collective action. That misplaced veneration propelled me to entertain a run for Congress with no knowledge of the actual job description—cramped rooms equipped only with a telephone and a list of names, some not entirely reputable. Unending supplications. Party discipline. Eroded principle. But there seemed no ceiling on my hunger for renown.

I was relatively young and chronically furious with our Republican congressmen, often debating them in noisy, indignant dreams. For years we had given money and written letters to the editor for a parade of Democratic candidates tilting at the windmills of Kansas' political landscape. But when a congressional seat opened in 2017, I asked then Senator Laura Kelly's advice on running. She urged instead that I support a stronger candidate who would soon announce.

Paul Davis definitely was that candidate, a prominent Lawrence lawyer with deep Kansas roots and a decade of experience in the state senate. Tall, reassuring. His opponent had no such experience, and a platform limited to more guns and fewer abortions. We gave money, hosted a reception, did background research, even appeared in a TV ad. We Topeka Democrats in the Ramada ballroom were euphoric on election night as the early returns came in. But the race tightened as the hours passed and the seat ultimately went to the bearer of the Republican brand.

I was forcefully reminded that night of where I lived and of how short my reach was; reminded of identity's power, the force of tribal belonging. I struggle even now to square those voters with the community that joined me in grief at my parents' death. But I would bet their world teemed with enemies, as mine had. That their identity, like mine, was an inheritance not easily eroded by argument.

Craig Yorke

In that darkened Ramada ballroom, I took refuge in a history of small actions. My friend Pedro honored me with his invitation to welcome about 100 new citizens at Topeka's federal district courthouse—the privilege to speak and to feel the force that had pulled them here. Helping to send two Yorke scholars to college each year. Walking our leafy neighborhood to get out the vote as Democratic precinct committee person. Celebrating the citizens our sons have become. Elections come and go, but I've come to see our days as filled with political acts, each minutely shifting the polis for good or ill, acts possible for each of us. This was a new way to see, a new way to occupy the space "between the world and me," to see karma defined—each action having its result. Today those memories ground me as the shrill voices of cable news toggle us between rage and fear.

Raising our sons was a daily political act, among other things. We shielded them from want and, imperfectly, from bigotry. There were language camps, music lessons, backcountry treks. Foreign exchange students like Yoko Kobayashi enlivened our prairie home. Her English at its most primitive ran rings around our Japanese and her courtesy was almost stereotypical as she tried to make sense of two noisy boys and a noisy nation. She offered them (and us) a glimpse of the world.

But affluence carries its own hazards and civilizing our adolescent boys was a major challenge. Their late-night misadventures at Topeka High gave us more than our share of gray hairs. Pride flipped to shame, denting my ancient and fragile self-image more than once. Mercifully, their errors were nonfatal, and a new peer group magically appeared as they entered the 11th grade. I couldn't replicate the desperation of Corey Road. I kept my thumb off their future's scale, hoping my own life would persuade more clearly than any angry admonition. As Mary and I sat at our kitchen table well past their curfew, resolving every few minutes not to look at the wall clock, I instead stared at the wall, frozen in uncertainty. But this was not Corey Road. A large house, but in one way smaller. It had little room for "big people," so we grew to be heroes by default.

Mary often shouldered the role of bad cop on those nights. I was tired, and timid. I feared I'd become my dad, my fears spiraling into hard words. My motives were mixed, tangled. But I did show up, day after day. And the boys did come through those years with judgment and resilience that have served them well. I had grown just big enough to glimpse a wider perspective, to loosen history's grip a fraction and rebut Faulkner's words about the past—had grown small enough to step back and win a hint of freedom for myself. The boys were both art majors in college. We worried how they'd support themselves, but they paid their own price and landed on their feet. And each day their mind's educated eyes see the world in ways few of us can imagine.

They feel the force of their own history today, but they've been able to choose their own paths in ways I couldn't, and have been recognized for their own gifts. They had little need for my armor. Zack took a winding path through Watson and Fulbright fellowships in South Africa, then detoured briefly for a suit and tie corporate stint. He's landed at Google as a researcher. Chris became an architect and took on projects around the world, from retail stores to treehouses, and eventually opened his own design studio. They've both enlisted their skills to serve their imagination. And they're both more attentive dads than I ever was. They enrich my world and temper my fear of senescence as they carry our DNA into our species' unknowable future. And they're my best evidence that I've won a taste of freedom from my past.

Our family huddled together in the bleachers against the unseasonable cold of early June 2004. My rear end was losing heat to the aluminum plank at an uncomfortable pace. We family and friends had been issued identical purple ponchos against the light rain. One size did indeed fit all. They'd been freshly picked from their packaging that morning and gave us all a potent smell of virgin vinyl. They carried the seal of Williams College. We'd come for Chris' class day and graduation. He had shown us around and Dad, now 89, was delighted to remember his electrical design work on the college's Clark Museum.

The cold prolonged the wait. Our program assured us that the graduates would soon march into the stadium in alphabetical order in their caps and gowns. The band struck up the school song. The ground fog broke a bit, and we glimpsed the stars of the show moving in our direction. A banner flew at their head. Its bearer was tall, difficult to make out but somehow familiar. Whoa! It was Chris, unleashed from the "Ys" at the rear of the procession! The artist, the dreamer, carrying the class flag he'd designed—our resilient kid, much loved at whatever end of this happy parade he appeared.

He and Susan had first met in sophomore math class. Williamstown is a small place, and the students saw lots of each other. Now their cautious romance had bloomed. They would marry on the shore of Lake Crescent in Olympic National Park. This gorgeous venue introduced urban kids to the natural world during the week and covered the expense by hosting weekend weddings. I was to help with the music—time to pull out the fiddle and brush up on Wagner's wedding march. We'd never been to the Olympic. It's one of the less visited parks, probably because it's not particularly on the way to anywhere else.

Mary and I drove three hours north and west from Seattle, presented our lifetime entry pass at the park's southern gate. We were the only car in sight. We noticed an absence of signage and turnouts, pulled onto a narrow shoulder, and parked. We were abruptly alone as we wandered down an overgrown trail. This rain forest was immensely dense, the smell of its earth ancient but entirely new to me. The Sequoias erased the sky, some reaching 300 feet into the air. Many generations of leaves and needles cushioned our every step.

Time ran in reverse, sprinted millennia in that moment. It's said in the Thomas Gospel that the kingdom of heaven is spread upon the earth, but men do not see it. This forest would have been invisible to young Craig and even now revealed only a glimpse of itself. But on this day the student was more ready, and the teacher briefly appeared. Such a parade of growth and life, decay and death. Infinite shades of green, unnumbered plants I had no hope of naming. We stood at the childhood of the world, suspended in that instant between past and future.

The newlyweds' honeymoon destination was a mystery. Chris casually mentioned at the reception that they would spend their next year in Palau, she as an advisor to their supreme court, he as a residential architect. We were speechless. We knew it was a Pacific island but that didn't help us much in locating it. They invited us to visit and didn't have to ask twice.

We laid over in Tokyo, then four hours south to Guam. Finally, Palau. Full-on tropical heat, weighty air, daily afternoon monsoon. The Japanese had defended the island group in the battle of Peleliu, though few Americans could now recall the name and fewer could locate the place on a map. Nearly 10,000 U.S. Marines and an equal number of Japanese had been wounded or killed there during 21 days of autumn in 1944, in what was decorously understated as a campaign of island hopping.

Palau is also among the most famous diving spots in the world. I'd taken up scuba in retirement but had made only a few dives. Chris and Susan dove several times each week and were well on their way to the muscle memory of unconscious expertise. The German channel was a storied site and did not disappoint—a blizzard of unnamable fish, a riot of color. The cheapest ticket to an alien planet and cause for awe, shrinking the biggest of us if we have eyes to see.

As we descended past 50 feet, the world became more blue. A manta ray slid by just a foot over my head, briefly blocking the already dimmed sun. The flat eyes of sharks almost my size registered my bubbles as they went on their way. Sherlock was our divemaster and guide. The name suggested 19th century London, but he was very much Palauan, large enough to try his hand at Sumo. He tossed our tanks around as though they were weightless and guided our boat to and from the channel, pointing out various landmarks and subtleties of color and swell on what to me was a perfectly featureless expanse of ocean.

A few days later we did an easier dive to a more somber place. At a spot only 100 yards from shore we found a Japanese Zero, its dreaded fighter plane, almost perfectly preserved in 30 feet of water. It was home to a crowd of busy fish and a serene coffin for a drafted youngster. My bubbles ascended but my mind stopped. The world was more complex than Corey Road's assurances. A few shore batteries still stood watch over the coast, mostly around the harbor. Unexploded ordnance littered the island. An Australian NGO would disarm it over the next several years. The U.S. Marines had expected token resistance. Bob Hope had wished them well the night before the battle began. Japan had lost that ferocious fight in 1944, but its hotels and car dealerships had since won the island back. And it was time for us to head back to Tokyo.

We had packed thoroughly both for tropical diving and for urban exploration. Our former foreign exchange student, Yoko Kobayashi, by now a realtor and mother, was ready to welcome us. I'd written out about 20 Japanese survival phrases on a 3x5 card and had been practicing on the flight. We boarded a high-speed train at Narita airport for the central downtown Tokyo rail station and got off with some confidence and lots of luggage. We emerged into a surging maelstrom of black-suited salarymen racing in every possible direction. Picture Grand Central Station at rush hour, totally jammed with unsmiling young men. The Japanese signage was distant and not well lit. And there were no words on those signs, only characters. *Hiragana*? *Katakana*? So much for my index card. So much for my treasured competence. We couldn't move. We certainly couldn't speak. I had a rogue thought that we were perfectly good enough right on this spot and leaked a tiny laugh, but quickly suppressed it. It would come more easily today. The crush of humanity was intense, and no words of English were to be heard. Even had we known which way to go, our baggage immobilized us. No daylight or stairs were visible. We were misplaced, foreigners, *gaijin* by definition.

After a brief eternity, a young man attached to a weighty leather briefcase paused to take note of this novel obstacle to his commute.

His soft eyes met ours. He looked out over the sea of humanity and gently set down his case, then used a bit of sign language to point us in the direction of the lights of a distant elevator. After several bows and earnest *arigatos* we set off. Once we'd reached it, we and our bags hesitated to occupy too much of its modest space but managed to clamber on. I glanced at the numbers on the buttons, pulled out my index card, and noted that we were seven stories below ground. So, there was some climbing to do, but now we did have a lift.

We took advantage of Chris' junior year abroad to visit him in Australia, but Dad fell ill with us halfway across the globe. He had been himself days before, relishing a pizza and sharing his wisdom with Zack in a biographic video interview. Now a head injury from a fall on the ice at his retirement community signaled his final illness. Zack suddenly became his next of kin, our keen eyes and ears. He told us to hurry home. We endured an endless flight from Sydney in 2005 to find Dad lethargic and struggling to speak in a far too familiar ICU. He'd done amazingly well after a similar trauma four years earlier, but now was sleepy and struggled with the tenacious secretions of COPD. He couldn't speak a sentence, his right leg nearly flaccid. As is typical, the advance directives he'd crafted so carefully didn't address his specific situation. But this was a man who lived to talk and to move.

I waited. And waited. I wept, finally sought help from hospice. I so wanted him to stay with me, but my love for him had grown up a little and I prayed it could flower in memory. His pneumonia was quick, the morphine a mercy. His death was less sudden than Mom's, my state of mind a bit more prepared for pain and loss.

He had bounced through several addresses and jobs after Mom's death. His second marriage was brief and unhappy, undertaken in haste by a grieving man. But he cherished special lady friends until his end. He was proud of his son although I hadn't become a professor or flown my own jet, even more proud of his grandsons. Many Topekans loved him, blissfully unaware of the demons beefing and jostling for headroom just behind his beaming smile.

He and Mom did much with what they had. They far exceeded America's expectations, were unlikely patriots. They found hope in the unseen and raised a son for a future they had no reason to welcome. The Enlightenment's brand-new message of "created equal" grounded their citizenship, however much Jefferson might have despised them. And the gift of the civil rights movement contained the assignment of creating a more perfect union, beginning at our kitchen table. Their history carried immense force, and they acted heroically within it, even on their most desperate days. Their story made no news. They were no celebrities, but more than worthy of celebration. I had long admired them beyond words. On many days I believe I've acted well too, well enough even to justify their sacrifice. And by now I've grown or shrunk enough to feel a new love for them, not because of their heroics. Just because.

Because I'd been schooled to succeed invisibly, even a former patient's friendly greeting at the grocery store was vaguely unsettling. To be singled out for a major award was a shock. In 2014 St. Francis Hospital honored Mary and me with their Caritas Award as the city's outstanding medical couple. We young lovers in the faded foreign car had built an honorable life in an unlikely place, were no longer fledgling pillars in this community. The ranks of my enemies had thinned.

The award carried its moment of fruition but felt far different than I'd imagined. I worried, of course, about what to wear and what to say. I reached for my seventh grade Latin dictionary and learned that the word caritas means "caring" today, but long ago it meant "possessing value." Value became my theme, and value was what we'd created over those 35 years. The banquet food was forgettable and my speech too long, but friends' and family's presence, physical and virtual, meant the world.

I served on several boards over those years and consistently hated asking people for money. I was skillful but my reluctance grew more intense with time. Perpetual fundraising for struggling nonprofits was an unwelcome reminder of my gritty past. I took the struggle personally, and so also the anxiety and the pain.

But the Kansas Children's Discovery Center was different. It was 2009 and Topeka, along with only three other state capitals, had no children's museum. We on the founding board set out to change that. We launched a $6 million capital campaign, the largest in the city's history, into the trough of a historic recession. An effort five years earlier had failed, and we were less likely to succeed.

I learned lots about architecture, city politics, and early childhood development during that campaign, but mostly I learned about fundraising in hard times. Topeka's brand as "a good place to raise kids" did open a few grandparents' wallets. And the idea of outdoor "serious" fun as a vehicle to promote fitness, scientific thinking, and the natural world began to take hold. We were working with vacant acreage in a city park. Chris and I walked the site in midwinter. As we scouted likely trees for the treehouse he'd later design and build, we surprised a coyote in the brush. It regarded us for an instant and vanished without a sound.

Mary chose part of the site south of the Center to honor her parents with a pollinator garden and conceived the idea of a tallgrass prairie restoration to surround it. We opened in 2011. I was a beginner and brought that mind to the effort. The work was fun because its goal was concrete, because I learned so much—and of course, because we succeeded. Whenever I return with our own grandkids I relish the ceiling, the use of light, the space itself. I'm reminded of the design debates and budgeting struggles behind every detail of its architecture, and I'm glad that we could improve our town. The pollinator garden has thrived and, if history holds, the prairie restoration will long outlive the building.

In 2003, I reintroduced myself to my fiddle. I'm surprised Mary didn't move out, because those first couple of years were excruciating. It had to have been the invisible noise canceling buds she'd secreted in her ears. I'd warred against the instrument as a kid, had seen it as an enemy. Now after 35 years I slowly came to see a few of its multiple personalities—talisman of parental love, unlikely heirloom, wooden box of rare beauty.

I remember the pain of the Gardner Museum well but no longer suffer with it. I pay full attention to that old fiddle each day. The fingertips of my left hand have reacquired their calluses but the cuts that troubled me as a kid haven't returned. I've unyoked from the instrument to embrace it, to focus while relaxing, and make daily practice into a meditation. Less has become more.

Tennis has become meditative too. Focusing on a fuzzy lime-green sphere absorbs attention. I do love the game—to move on the court, to attend to the ball's rotation, to hear my shoes squeak on the asphalt. I played competitively for a few years and had some success in my cohort of old guys. I played with fellow boomers at a national tournament in Indian Wells, California and swear that walking onto those royal blue courts channeled my secret touring pro—a step quicker, my club foot a relic of some distant past. But it's hitting with our sons that gives the most intense pleasure, all the more because that pleasure must be transient, just like me. I inhabit a miraculous machine, now 76 years old.

I was supremely confident as I packed for our hike in the Grand Canyon in February 2018. I knew what I was doing, knew what to expect. Our group of three old doctors, led by Ben Franklin, had gone rim-to-rim two years before in June. That had been a hot and trying trek. We'd made a steep descent from the South Rim, our thigh muscles complaining as we reached the banks of the Colorado River and set up camp near Phantom Ranch. We planned to leave for the North Rim the next morning. The ranger advised us to be gone before sunrise to avoid being caught in a nearby canyon, respectfully labeled "the box," after 10 a.m. The box had claimed the lives of a few hikers over the years, and I saw why in a couple of hours. The canyon was narrow, steep, and tall. Its walls were deep red, almost burgundy, and even with the June sun not fully overhead, the air temperature had reached triple digits. There was no way up the walls. We ventured up to the North Rim and retraced our steps back to our starting place, Mather Point. Our voyage of two ascents and descents had occupied a memorable week, had overflowed with delicious memories.

Ben told us that this time we'd take a more relaxed gentleman's stroll east on the Tonto Trail. It paralleled the Colorado river on the south side of the canyon, a bit more than halfway down to the canyon's base. 35 miles of relatively level terrain over one week. We'd be going in winter, but I fully trusted the weather forecast and reasoned that I could live with the fact that my sleeping bag was rated down only to 40 degrees. I looked at a true winter bag but rejected it in a moment of Filene's Basement frugality. I stocked up on freeze dried meals and saved weight in my backpack wherever I could. I was very much the expert.

The first sign of trouble came as we descended from the South Rim and reached our first camp. Snow. Not much, but also not forecast. To assume that the weather at the rim would have any relevance for the lower reaches of the canyon was clearly a mistake, but hardly fatal. The next morning, we set off east on the trail, which I found far more irregular and challenging than the map had suggested. We made good progress, but the cold left me chronically hungry. The air was still and pure, the beauty beyond my vocabulary. We were less than gnats on the landscape but felt we could belong in this sublime unforgiving place. The mornings were noiseless, the stillness broken only by the breaking of our camp. The canyon felt eternal although the geologists assured us it was not. "Everything that begins also ends," said the Buddha, including the canyon, and us. We talked about contingencies if one of us were injured or became ill. We agreed that major injury would be a fatal problem here. To reach the rim for help would simply take too long. The rangers knew our route, but we had no satellite radio. We had only one human encounter during that week, an older woman hiking west, superbly fit and well informed.

I had planned carefully, but now realized that each of my freeze dried "dinners" contained no more than 600 calories. Meanwhile the snow fell intermittently, maybe an inch or so at a time. The trail was still visible.

By day four I'd resorted to sleeping in my hiking clothes to retain heat. I'd not take them off for the next three days and nights. My groin began to chafe, then to burn. I assumed my skin was breaking down and widened my gait to compensate. Daytime highs were about 35, nights about 20. My gloves were not quite up to the cold, leaving me uncoordinated in the most basic tasks of meal prep and camp maintenance. Ben and Tim Allen skillfully assembled and broke down our stove for each dinner. I'd exhausted my water and refilled from a nearby spring, though the rangers had warned us that it contained traces of tritium.

By day five I'd reached the end of my provisions, but on day seven we'd also reached our point of ascent back to the South Rim. It seemed a steep but straightforward climb, although the morning's snow was just enough to obscure what was already a seldom-used trail. My pack weighed less than 30 pounds by now, but I'd saved weight in part by not packing crampons and now regretted that decision with each slip and setback. Tim and Ben had avoided that mistake.

We made multiple starts onto false trails, sliding back to our starting point while burning calories I couldn't afford. The occasional cairn of piled rocks left as guidance by earlier hikers made all the difference. I was grateful then and am grateful now for those thoughtful little stone pyramids. We all could use such cairns when life gets narrow and steep.

Visibility was probably 20 yards. My legs were still strong, but the cold was front of mind. We'd broken camp that morning at 8 and, as the weather cleared, we had our first glimpse of the South Rim at about 11. Like every landmark in the canyon, it was far more distant than it appeared. But seeing the destination shortened the path. We continued our climb as the snow let up and reached the rim at 2, a bit less than a mile of ascent in six hours. I gave thanks to my legs as they quivered in silent outrage. We were very much by ourselves in this sublime winter landscape, a celestial setting

STEEP

perfectly indifferent to hunger and cold more intense than I'd ever known.

We quickly found our rented vehicle and set off—and promptly encountered a livestock fence fixed across our only road out of the park. It was held shut by an enormous padlock, and the road was so severely crowned that going around it into the ditch would have been a serious mistake. Our gas tank was nearly full, and we fired up the heater. Our phones had no charge, but we plugged one into the 12-volt outlet and started looking through our documents for an emergency number. A recorded message told us that the park service had closed all roads due to weather conditions. We left a strained voicemail after the beep and wondered what would come next.

Miraculously, what came next after about 15 minutes was one of their vehicles appearing from nowhere. A smiling, bemused ranger said he'd just been passing by and unlocked the chain to let us escape to the closest motel.

I stuffed my hiking clothes into the motel's plastic laundry bag to enclose their stench and took the longest shower of my life, hoping that the eroded skin of my inner thighs would heal quickly, that the searing chafe would soon pass. No one would mistake me for a cowboy, but I walked like one for a week. I sidled up to the motel room's creaking baseboard heater and relished its smell of burning metal, then joined my partners at the all-you-can-eat buffet and inhaled at least 5,000 calories in 15 minutes, wordlessly grateful for the limitless refined sugar and saturated fat, for the gigantic indulgence brimming with unpronounceable additives. I slept long and well.

-8-
NEW EYES

The real voyage in discovery consists not in seeking new landscapes but in having new eyes.
—*Marcel Proust*

"We need more data," said my new internist. He scanned me with mournful, thorough eyes. My "bad" cholesterol had been high for 20 years, but I was relatively fit and had had no "events." We both knew that statin drugs helped prevent heart attacks and strokes in people with high cholesterol who'd already suffered them, but that no reliable statistics existed for folks like me.

"We need more data," he repeated, and scheduled a scan to measure how much calcium had been deposited in my coronary arteries over the previous seven decades. For an instant I regretted those many gallons of ice cream and protested that no treatment could possibly flow from any conceivable scan result. He gave me a tired smile, reminded me that the scan was noninvasive, the radiation exposure minimal, and that the cost of ignorance...well, I recalled my mom's end.

The scan ended before it began. As I got into my running shoes at home an hour later my phone lit up. "Your calcium score is more than triple the upper limits of normal. A panic value. Take an aspirin right now. Pick up the atorvastatin I've prescribed and start today. You see the cardiologist at 9 tomorrow."

I knew him well—about 50, skillful, attentive. His voice was chatty, his eyes urgent, his advice clear. Cardiac catheterization—soon—to define blocked arteries in need of stenting or bypass. He asked about my general state of health. His eyes widened when I volunteered that I ran without a cellphone. "No! No! Stop!" he said, feigning humor. "Can you imagine how I'd look if my patient, the retired neurosurgeon, is found dead on the Shunga Trail?"

My name reached the cath schedule in no time at all and we

journeyed to the hospital at sunrise. Mary suppressed her anxiety well. I aimed to be calm, but the scan was a preview of coming attractions for this aging man. I was prepped for open heart surgery—groins shaved, lines in place. I looked around the cath lab at all the gleaming machines I hoped wouldn't prove necessary and recalled the many ORs of my past. I wasn't today's performer, but would good enough mean robust health—or possibly survival? So, I'd trekked for decades to reach this destination, now seen as if for the first time. Supine on a metal slab surrounded by a squad of absurdly young strangers? I'd believed I was gliding down life's highway when in fact I might well be slip sliding away.

The propofol and fentanyl erased consciousness and time. I wakened to hear that I had calcium everywhere in my heart, but nowhere severe enough for treatment—and that I'd been blessed with plus-sized coronary vessels.

I counted each leaf of each tree as I wobbled to the car, the mind-altering drugs not fully cleared. I faced into the north wind, grateful for the moving air. I resolved to decalcify my heart, or at least to soften it, and was reminded that because life is short it's precious. So what we do matters. And that we do well to honor our past but do better to live our own lives well.

Awe can slip by stealth into our well-ordered minds to gift us new vision. It also can blow us out of the ruts of our daily life. It can overwhelm distraction and is the expert's enemy. It can open us to humility. But wonder doesn't spring from bargain hunting or from immersion in electronic images. And trotting the globe offers no guarantee because our past fits so comfortably into our luggage. But if we work to make ourselves eligible, if we can pay attention, the sublime will ambush us, can erase past and future and wake us to right now. With practice, even small surprises can do the same, and more often. Today I claim no special expertise. My tale unrolls over decades, is untweetable. It lacks glamour because it happens next door. But the story of someone like me (or you) insists that any of us can build an honorable life under imperfect circumstances.

STEEP

This little book began as a letter to our sons, to say what's nudged aside in the press of family gatherings. To look back has been a blessing. I've gained much from the effort but don't presume to instruct them or you. This is no sermon, only scenes from a life. I'm no victim and my words no invitation to outrage. I was forged to live in a world far more hostile than the one I've come to occupy, and maintaining balance in the face of such rapid change has been a trial. History's grip is strong, and its whisper of "not good enough" has echoed in endless variations through my years. It drove many praiseworthy actions but couldn't create a wholly selfless motive for any of them. My path has had ups and downs. I've found no shortcuts. But I've come to see more selves inside me—and so to be more free. And I've come to see my neighbors as not altogether bad or good, but as more or less unhappy, and so all in need of a good turn.

We all want our lives to make sense, want our heroes and villains to stay put, our armored selves fixed in virtue. Our past pulls us into a tribe and craves its victory. But the critical moments of our lives are lived alone, and in those moments tribal boundaries wobble, and we're pushed into an uncertain future. Topeka's peaks and valleys unstuck me a little, slowly gifted me a more fluid self, big or small at need—reminded me enough of my past to give our sons not freedom from pain or error, but a chance to realize themselves. Allowed me a glimpse of belonging and peace in this eighth decade of life.

Our very words tether us to ancient history, but also give us new language to see it. Two Sanskrit words, samsara and nirvana, come to mind. They translate into English usage as words of one syllable. Samsara means to move or to run, captures the distractions of our lives. Think of a perpetual treadmill or, if not perpetual, as permanent as a human life. And I did spend years running, aiming to create a bulletproof identity.

My reality today is different. Most of us experience our eighth decade as a time of loss. Loss of energy, of proper nouns and much else. A series of unwelcome, ultimately disabling events visited on us by our aging bodies. But we could instead embark consciously on a process of subtraction, of disarmament. Divesting layers of armor, loosening attachments to erudition or status. I intend to welcome that alternative, aspire to see the fires of my cravings slowly blown out, my attachments cooled off. Those little words—blown out, cooled off—convey the literal meaning of samsara's antonym, nirvana.

I punched my ticket and paid for success. The price was my childhood, its friendships and its daydreams, what might have been the arc of my identity in a more friendly world. I forfeited an American adolescence. Softer bits of myself were buried in the climb. The journey was not quick, not easy. The price was steep, its currency physical, cultural, intellectual. In return came eyes to see and fertile time to write. I was mined from a redlined 'hood and transplanted to an American pot nowhere near melting. For decades I lived the lives of others, 50 years as a surrogate, another 20 looking for an elusive self inside the role. I chased expertise and the clarity of the familiar.

Today I'm more at ease with my uncertain station in the scheme of things, more at ease with who I was and am, even with what I'll become. A fragile, welcome change. Serenity sneaks up on me at odd moments, bringing a kind of privilege, a privilege of time, honestly come by and free of color. And I have lived a full life. The grail of education offered me less a bigger name than a bigger perspective, a tortuous map away from the confines of a hard history. My bunker has grown, has made room for a skylight and picture windows. I've taken to heart that chiseled advice on Harvard Yard's gate, have aimed to grow in wisdom, am slower to name villains and fix blame. I can befriend that chubby kid on the subway with his leaden briefcase and distressed lunch bag. Can wish the Mr. McCormicks of the world well. Tallying debits and credits I'll leave to others, but to know that I've done what I could with what I had is a mercy.

Proust's new eyes don't come cheap or arrive by same-day delivery. History can wield paralyzing power but Baldwin's right that its force is unconscious. We best face it by waking up, by using what eyes we have to see it as it is, not as we wish or fear it to be. We make use of memory to nudge our cravings toward love, to inch our way toward liberation. Then we prisoners can win moments of parole, can welcome our ancient demons, and so soften their grip.

ACKNOWLEDGEMENTS

Steep. The adjective conjures a precipitous climb—or descent. But the verb connotes a ripening over time.

Many voices have ripened this story. Cy Console encouraged me to persist. I've aspired to use words as he does. Tom Averill broadened my vision and connected me with Thea Rademacher of Flint Hills Publishing. Her patience and skill have brought this work into your hands.

Early readers like Todd Fertig and Tim Russell clarified the writing. Bryant York fact checked the family history. Sam Potts reimagined the cover.

Nate Frederickson, my learned and boisterous editor, pushed me to rearrange the chronology. His wisdom brought this narrative to life.

Finally—family. Chris reminded me more than once to find pleasure in all this steeping, then proceeded to nail the cover's design. Zack somehow created time to know the text as well as I do. His eye for coherence and modern usage erased many shortcomings. And Mary was, and is, the last best voice in my head, the ground from which this story emerges. More than my better half.

Steep's strengths flow from this team. Any errors are mine.

ABOUT THE AUTHOR

Craig Yorke was born in Roxbury, Massachusetts. He received a BA from Harvard College and an MD from Harvard Medical School. After residency training at the University of California San Francisco, he practiced neurosurgery in Topeka, Kansas for nearly 25 years. He lives in Topeka and makes coffee each morning for his wife, Mary. Their two sons are a blessing. He is a credible violinist and hits tennis balls with passion. *Steep* is his first book.

www.craigyorke.com

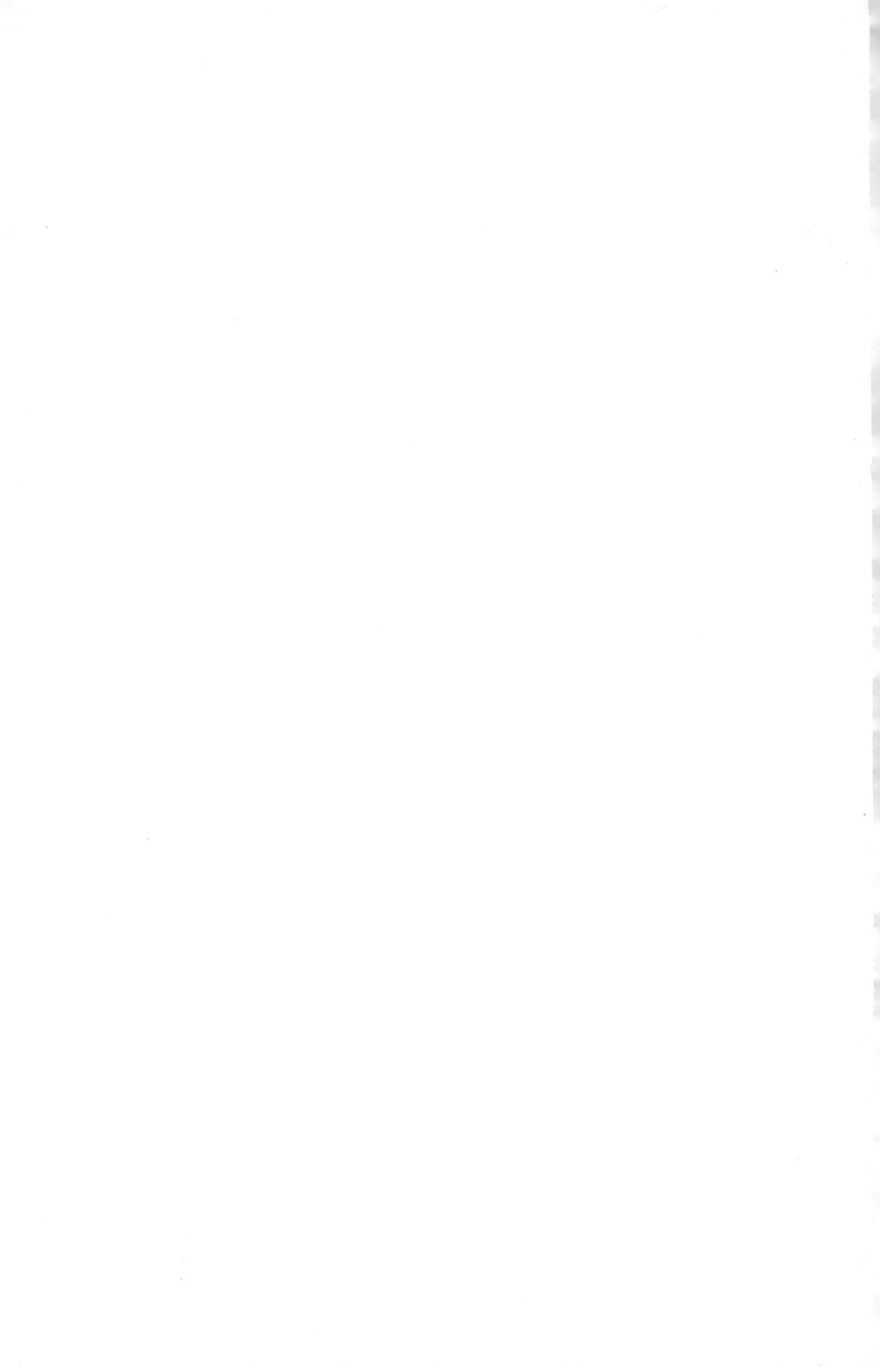